Primary Biliary Cirrhosis:
From Pathogenesis to Clinical Treatment

Primary Biliary Cirrhosis:
From Pathogenesis to Clinical Treatment

Edited by

Keith D. Lindor
Professor of Medicine
Mayo Clinic
200 First Street SW
Rochester, MN 55905
USA

E. Jenny Heathcote
Professor of Medicine
University of Toronto
The Toronto Hospital, Western Division
399 Bathurst Street, Wing 4-828
Toronto, ONT M5T 2S8
Canada

Raoul Poupon
Professor of Medicine
Service d'Hepatologie et Gastroenterologie
AP – Hôpital Saint-Antoine
184, rue Du Faubourg, Saint-Antoine
75571 Paris
France

The proceedings of a symposium organised by AXCAN PHARMA,
held in Chicago, November 6, 1997

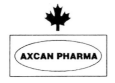

KLUWER ACADEMIC PUBLISHERS
DORDRECHT / BOSTON / LONDON

Library of Congress Cataloging-in-Publication Data

A C.I.P. Catalogue record for this book is available from the Library of Congress.

ISBN 0-7923-8740-6

Published by Kluwer Academic Publishers PV,
PO Box 17, 3300 AA Dordrecht, The Netherlands.

Sold and distributed in North, Central and South America
by Kluwer Academic Publishers, PO Box 358,
Accord Station, Hingham, MA 02018-0358, USA

In all other countries, sold and distributed
by Kluwer Academic Publishers, Distribution Centre,
PO Box 322, 3300 AH Dordrecht, The Netherlands

Printed on acid-free paper

Printed in Great Britain.

Contents

CONTENTS

Scientific Organizers

KEITH D. LINDOR
Professor of Medicine
Mayo Clinic
200 First Street SW
Rochester, MN 55905
USA

E. JENNY HEATHCOTE
Professor of Medicine
University of Toronto
Chief, Division of Gastroenterology
The Toronto Hospital, Western Division
399 Bathurst Street, Wing 4-828
Toronto, ONT M5T 2S8
Canada

RAOUL POUPON
Professor of Hepatology and Gastroenterology
Department of Pathology
AP – Hôpital Saint-Antoine
184, rue Du Faubourg
75571 Paris
France

List of Principal Authors

M. F. BASSENDINE
Liver Unit
Freeman Hospital
Newcastle upon Tyne
NE7 7DN
UK

N. V. BERGASA
Division of Gastroenterology & Liver Disease
Beth Israel Medical Center
First Avenue at 16th Street
New York
NY 10003
USA

R. L. CARITHERS Jr.
Hepatology Section
University of Washington
1959 NE Pacific Street
Seattle
WA 98195-0004
USA

E. R. DICKSON
Division of Gastroenterology and Hepatology
Mayo Clinic (W19)
200 First Street SW
Rochester
MN 55905
USA

J. EVERHART
Epidemiology and Clinical Trials Branch
Division of Digestive Diseases and Nutrition
National Institute of Diabetes and Digestive and Kidney Diseases
Natcher Building, Room 6AN-12J
45 Center Dr MSC 6600
Bethesda MD 20892-6600
USA

M. E. GERSHWIN
University of California at Davis
Division of Rheumatology, Allergy and Clinical Immunology
One Shields Avenue, TB 192, School of Medicine
Davis CA 95616-8660
USA

C. D. HOWELL
Hepatology Section
The University of Maryland School of Medicine
22 S Green St Room N3W 130
Baltimore
MD 21201-1595
USA

P.-M. HUET
Hepatology Research Group
CHUM Clinical Research Center
Saint-Luc Pavillon
164 René-Lévesque Blvd. E.
Montreal
QC H2X 1P1
Canada

O. F. W. JAMES
School of Clinical Medical Sciences
University of Newcastle
Senior Consultant Physician
Liver Unit
Freeman Hospital
Newcastle upon Tyne
NE2 4HH
UK

R. JOPLIN
Liver Research Laboratories
University Hospital
The Queen Elizabeth Hospital
Birmingham
B15 2TH
UK

M. M. KAPLAN
Tufts University School of Medicine
Gastroenterology Division
New England Medical Center
750 Washington Street, Box 233
Boston
MA 02111
USA

R. KLEIN
Department of Internal Medicine
University of Tübingen
Otfried Müller Str. 10
72076 Tübingen
Germany

J. NEUBERGER
The Liver Unit and Hepatobiliary Unit
The Queen Elizabeth Hospital
Birmingham
B15 2TN
UK

A. PARÉS
Liver Unit
Hospital Clinic i Provincial
Calle Villarroel 170
08036 Barcelona
Spain

G. PAUMGARTNER
Department of Medicine II
Klinikum Grosshadern
Marchioninistrasse 15
D-81377 Munich
Germany

J. PRIETO
Department of Medicine and Liver Unit
Clínica Universitaria de Navarra
Avenida Pio XII, 36
E-31008 Pamplona
Spain

D. SCHUPPAN
Department of Medicine I (Gastroenterology & Hepatology)
University of Erlangen-Nürnberg
Krankenhausstr. 12
D-91054 Erlangen
Germany

M. G. SWAIN
Liver Unit, Gastroenterology Research Group
Health Sciences Center
University of Calgary
3330 Hospital Drive NW
Calgary
AB T2N 4N1
Canada

LIST OF PRINCIPAL AUTHORS

H. R. VAN BUUREN
Department of Hepatogastroenterology and Internal Medicine
University Hospital Rotterdam
Dr Molewaterplein 40
3015 GD Rotterdam
The Netherlands

J. M. VIERLING
Center for Liver Diseases and Transplantation
8635 West Third Street, Site 590W
Los Angeles
CA 90048
USA

Preface

The condition of prolonged obstructive jaundice with patent bile ducts was first described in 1851 by Addison and Gull of Guy's Hospital, London. The term primary biliary cirrhosis (PBC) was defined in 1950 by Ahrens and colleagues of the Rockefeller Institute, New York. The condition was considered rare but this changed in 1965 with the discovery of a definitive diagnostic serum mitochondrial antibody test and the recognition that a raised serum alkaline phosphatase value, often discovered incidentally, could be a diagnostic pointer. If the diagnosis is made earlier, the end stages are rarely reached as death is replaced by liver transplantation.

On November 6th 1997, in Chicago, an International Faculty discussed in depth the clinical features, pathogenesis and treatment of PBC, no longer considered a rare disease. The course of PBC is long, but some 18 years after the discovery of a positive mitochondrial antibody test in a symptom-free patient with normal serum biochemistry, 83% will have developed abnormal tests and 76% will be symptomatic. Identification of those who will progress rapidly is difficult. The serum antimitochondrial profile may be useful but this is a very specialist technique. Mathematical prognostic models are useful in therapeutic trials and in the selection and timing of patients for liver transplantation but have limited value in individual patients. An increasing serum bilirubin level remains the most important indicator of rapid progression. Its value however can be negated by the use of ursodeoxycholic acid which has a bilirubin-lowering effect.

PBC is generally considered to be an autoimmune disease. The sufferer is believed to be genetically predisposed. There is a weak association with MHC class II allele HLA DR8. The link is however not nearly so close as that found with autoimmune chronic active hepatitis.

The part played by mitochondrial antibodies (AMA) in pathogenesis remains controversial. The mitochondrial antigen responsible for the AMA is the pyruvate dehydrogenase complex (PDC). In PBC, aberrant expression of the E2 component of PDC has been shown on bile duct epithelium, possibly rendering bile ducts susceptible to immune-mediated damage. Alternatively, the disease may have an infectious etiology as there is cross-reactivity between AMA and sub-cellular constituents of Gram-positive and

Gram-negative organisms. The AMA found in PBC may be primarily directed against enterobacterial antigens resulting from intestinal infection.

The immunological lesion is mediated by CD4 T-cells secreting T-helper cytokines (IL-2, IFNγ, TNFα/β). Later, as the bile ducts disappear, fibrosis and cirrhosis develop. Cholestasis is enhanced by decreased levels of biliary transport proteins secondary to the biliary obstruction and to endotoxaemia.

Therapy can be directed against any of these injurious processes. Immunological manipulations have been many. Corticosteroids block CD4 lymphocytes but bone thinning prevents their long-term use. Azathioprine, chlorambucil, D-penicillamine and cyclosporin have been tested and generally found wanting, usually because of side-effects or failure to prove benefit in long-term placebo-controlled clinical trials. It is also difficult to justify the continued use, over many years, of drugs which have potential toxicity. Drug failures may also be related to the stage of the disease. It is clearly not possible to reverse cirrhotic nodules and fibrosis or the interference with hepatobiliary transport.

Colchicine, which has anti-inflammatory and anti-fibrotic actions, failed to provide conclusive benefit. Methotrexate may benefit some patients in the early stages of PBC but pneumonitis and hematological complications can develop. Ursodeoxycholic acid (UDCA; ursodiol) is currently the most effective medical therapy for PBC. Biochemical tests improve, progression of portal hypertension is reduced and time to death or liver transplantation is prolonged. However, histological changes in the liver progress and effects on lethargy and pruritus are variable. UDCA should be given to all symptomatic patients. The role in pre- and asymptomatic sufferers is not clear. The mechanism of action of UDCA is complex. The bile acid pool becomes more hydrophilic and less detergent so acting as a protectant of the luminal membrane of the interlobular bile ducts. UDCA stimulates the biliary excretion of endogenous hydrophobic (toxic) bile acids, perhaps by stimulating vesicular exocytosis by which transport carrier proteins are targeted to the canalicular membrane. Finally, UDCA may reduce the immune attack of cytotoxic T-cells by decreasing HLA1 expression on bile ducts.

Combinations of drugs may have greater benefit than monotherapy. UDCA plus methotrexate or corticosteroids is being assessed. Triple therapy with prednisolone, azathioprine and UDCA are under trial and results are awaited.

Fibrosis accompanies bile ductular proliferation and is responsible for the end picture of cirrhosis. Fibrosis is unaffected by immunomodulation or UDCA and holds the key to reversibility. This has led to therapy with such drugs as colchicine, silimarin and pentoxifyllin, which are largely ineffective. Better anti-fibrotic agents are awaited.

Complications such as ascites and portal hypertension need to be treated. Bone thinning may be reduced by etidronate and fluoride. Opiate antagonists are being used to control pruritus.

Hepatic transplantation performed before the terminal stages offers a five-year survival exceeding 85%. There is increasing evidence of recurrence in the graft. Granulomatous cholangitis develops in the livers of patients having a transplant for PBC but not where the operation is done for other indications. Short- and medium-term significance of the recurrence is probably little but longer follow-up is necessary.

The conference demonstrated the advantages of attracting international experts from various disciplines, clinical, immunological, biochemical, genetic and histopathological, to focus down on one disease. PBC, however, has something for everyone. It provides examples of model situations which can be applied to all of hepatology and indeed to all of general medicine.

Sheila Sherlock
Department of Surgery
Royal Free Hospital
London

Section I
Natural history and pathogenesis

1
Natural history and demography of primary biliary cirrhosis

O. F. W. JAMES

It will be impossible to deal at length with both the full natural history and demography of primary biliary cirrhosis in this short space. This will, therefore, be a review in three parts. The first will examine what we know about the early natural history of PBC and is intended to be read in conjunction with Chapter 9 by W. R. Kim and E. R. Dickson on Natural History Models of Primary Biliary Cirrhosis which will focus on the later clinical course of the disease. The second part will be a brief critical review of what we know of the world-wide distribution of PBC. In the third part, the preliminary results of a major case-finding study of the epidemiology of PBC in north-eastern England will be described. This will include information about the presentation and natural history of 770 patients, prevalent and incident, in a strict geographical area between the years 1987 and 1994 with follow-up data for a median of 6.3 years.

NATURAL HISTORY

Evidence concerning the earliest part of the natural history of PBC is derived from our studies of patients with positive antimitochondrial antibodies (AMA), measured by indirect immunofluorescence, who have been detected at a time when they had no abnormality of conventional liver function tests and no symptoms suggestive of liver disease. In 1986, we reported 29 patients with positive AMA (titer 1 in 40 or greater), normal conventional LFTs and no symptoms of liver disease. Liver histology was diagnostic of or compatible with PBC in 24 (83%) of these, and normal in only 2[1]. Seven of these 29 patients had been referred to the liver clinic for investigation of an incidental finding of positive AMA during investigations for other diseases. The other 22 were found by a review of all antibody screen results at the Northern Regional Immunology Laboratory to seek individuals with positive AMA (titer ≥ 1 in 40). These patients have now been followed up for 10 years following the original study[2]. The case records of all 29 patients were examined; all had been reviewed at annual intervals since 1985 or until death. Information on cause of death was obtained from death certificates and medical records. All surviving patients were interviewed and clinical and laboratory data recorded. Repeat liver biopsy samples were taken when clinically indicated.

The median total follow-up in these patients was 17.8 years (11–24 years). Twenty-four (83%) developed persistently abnormal LFTs and 22 (76%) developed typical symptoms of PBC (persistent severe lethargy and tiredness, pruritus, persistent right upper abdominal discomfort). Five patients died (median age 78): none died of liver disease although 2 had developed symptoms attributable to PBC. The median time from first positive AMA test to persistently abnormal liver blood tests was 5.6 years (0.9–19).

Repeat liver histology was available for 10 patients, a median of 11.4 years (1.33–14.3) after the original biopsies. In 9 patients, both original and follow-up biopsies were diagnostic of or compatible with PBC (assessed by a 'blinded' independent pathologist); in 1 patient, both biopsy samples were normal even after the development of slightly raised alkaline phosphatase and γ-GT. In this patient, the AMA titer had fallen to 1 in 20 and ELISA for the E2 components of pyruvate dehydrogenase complex and 2-oxoglutarate dehydrogenase complex was negative. Progress of histological stage was found in 4 of the 9 patients whose biopsy samples were diagnostic of or compatible with PBC.

Original baseline serum from 27 patients was available for testing by ELISA for the E2 components of PDC and 2-OGDC including all 24 patients who were alive at the follow-up review. In 21 patients, a positive ELISA was obtained from original and follow-up serum. All of these patients had original liver biopsy samples diagnostic of or compatible with PBC. Of the 6 ELISA-negative patients (ELISA negative on both original and follow-up serum samples), 1 had an original biopsy sample compatible with PBC; this patient subsequently developed pruritus, persistent lethargy, pain in the upper right quadrant, Sjögren's syndrome and hepatomegaly together with cholestasis. She refused further liver biopsy. This patient may be positive for branched chain oxoglutarate dehydrogenase complex as reported in about 5% of PBC cases.

The progression of PBC in our cohort was slow, even after the development of symptoms. Nonetheless, I believe that these studies have very clearly demonstrated that the vast majority of individuals with persistent markedly raised AMA (particularly if this is examined by ELISA) do have very early PBC and will sooner or later go on to develop clinical disease. We do not know whether development of AMA coincides with initiation of PBC or whether any external influences are involved in the pathogenesis of clinical PBC once AMA have appeared. Conceivably, as Lindor has suggested, some of these patients may form a subgroup, within the spectrum of PBC as a whole, who have a rather benign disease[3]. It is possible that patients with more 'progressive' or 'aggressive' disease pass through the phase of merely being AMA positive more quickly with the development of abnormal LFTs and symptoms over a shorter time frame.

As long ago as 1977, it was recognized that patients with positive AMA and cholestatic liver blood tests, but with no symptoms of liver disease, had

PBC[4]. Several groups have provided evidence concerning the natural history of such asymptomatic patients with abnormal LFTs, including our own report of 95 patients[5] and studies from the Mayo[6] and Yale[7]. In the joint Newcastle/Kings study[5], 95 initially asymptomatic patients were followed for a median 6 years. Thirty-four (36%) developed symptoms of liver disease; 15 of these died liver-related deaths. Survival in these 34 became identical to 277 other patients from the two centers who had been symptomatic at initial presentation. No predictors were found as to which of the 95 would develop symptoms although a higher proportion of those from Kings developed symptoms, and significantly more quickly, suggesting that, for whatever reason, referral to an international tertiary center might in some way influence the apparent natural history of these patients.

In the Mayo Clinic study[6], 73 initially asymptomatic patients were followed for a median 7.8 years. However, full follow-up data were only available in 44 of these. Symptoms developed in 33 (75%). Twelve of the 73 died of liver failure. Survival of this group was the same as an age-matched population at 6 years but subsequently was reduced compared with the age-matched control population up to 12 years follow-up (although numbers were by this time very small). The 36 patients from the Yale study[7] were followed for a median 12 years. One third of patients had developed symptoms by 6 years, two thirds by 12 years. Median survival for these initially asymptomatic patients was 16 years against 7.5 years for a group of 243 initially symptomatic patients from the same center. Again, overall survival of initially asymptomatic patients was shorter than the age-matched normal population but this difference only appeared after 11 years; again very small numbers were involved.

We can conclude that about 40% of initially asymptomatic PBC patients who have positive AMA and cholestatic liver blood tests with compatible or diagnostic histology will develop symptoms within 6 years. Once symptoms develop, survival is the same as for other symptomatic patients and can be estimated using the established Mayo model. In general, it is, at present, impossible to predict which of these initially asymptomatic patients will subsequently develop symptoms.

This information about the early natural history of the disease should inform our attitude to treatment. Current perception of this phase of the illness is summarized in Figure 1.

DEMOGRAPHY OF PBC

Descriptive epidemiology is the essential research tool with which to explore possible temporal and geographic variations in the frequency of PBC and thus to generate and test hypotheses about its cause. The epidemiology of PBC was not studied until Hamlyn and Sherlock's review of PBC deaths using death certification in England and Wales in 1974[8]. Since that time, a number of studies of the prevalence and incidence of PBC, largely from Europe, but more recently from Australia and Canada, have been described. We have recently carried out a critique of the methodology of these studies and examined the reasons for the poor quality of information contained

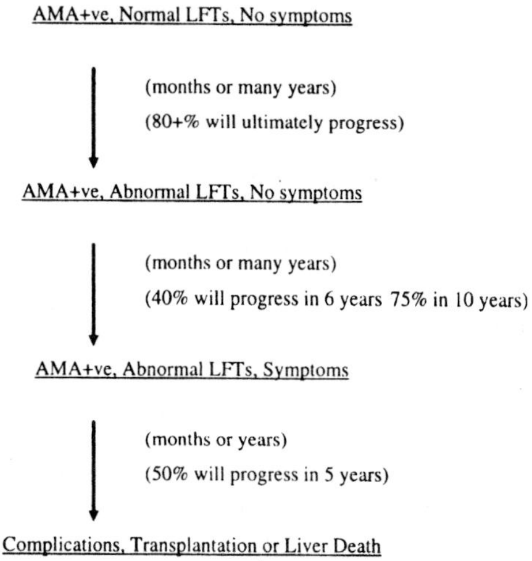

AMA+ve, Normal LFTs, No symptoms

(months or many years)
(80+% will ultimately progress)

AMA+ve, Abnormal LFTs, No symptoms

(months or many years)
(40% will progress in 6 years 75% in 10 years)

AMA+ve, Abnormal LFTs, Symptoms

(months or years)
(50% will progress in 5 years)

Complications, Transplantation or Liver Death

Figure 1 Natural history of PBC. NB. Because this is largely a disease of middle age and beyond, about half the patients will die of causes unrelated to liver disease.

within them and the lack of comparability between the studies[9]. It is perhaps not surprising that many studies, published up to 20 years ago, can be criticized today since epidemiology, like molecular biology, has made enormous recent advances in methodology. The problems with earlier studies may be summarized as follows:

1. Inconsistencies and lack of clarity in case definition.
2. Lack of precision in definition of the study area, population, and also the time period of study.
3. Incomplete case-finding methods.
4. Imprecision in the date of diagnosis.

Effectively, many studies have been case series in which the numbers of patients in the case series have been divided by the local population to give an estimate of prevalence.

In northern England, the prevalence of PBC has increased steadily over the past 20 years from $16/10^6$ in 1976 to $251/10^6$ in 1994 (Figure 2). Unfortunately, it is very hard to know what proportion of this increase is attributable to a true rise in prevalence and to what extent it is merely due to increasing awareness of the disease, increased diagnostic activity (particularly use of AMA testing) and to case finding. Certainly, our earlier case-finding studies fulfilled only some of the criteria for full case finding. These were fulfilled in our most recent study whose preliminary results are reported here. A summary of information concerning worldwide demography of PBC is presented in Table 1. An assessment of the 'quality' of the information is provided. No reliable information is available from Australasia, Asia or Africa. Other studies are graded: *, **, *** (best available). A fuller critique and references may be found in our recent review[9].

Table 1 Demography of PBC

Continent	Country	Prevalence/10^6	Quality
N. America	Canada	22	*
Europe	Sweden 1)	128	*
	2)	151	**
	England 1)	153	**
	2)	251	***
	EASL (1984)	5–75	—
	Estonia	27	*
Australasia	Australia	19	*
Asia	Japan	Case series suggest 'not uncommon'	
	India	Almost unknown	
Africa		No information: a few cases in whites	

Despite all the above comments, it is my strong anecdotal impression that prevalence is rising quite dramatically in a number of countries.

NORTH-EAST ENGLAND STUDY

We have recently completed a comprehensive case-finding study of the prevalence and incidence of PBC between 1 January 1987 and 31 December 1994 (followed until 31 December 1996) in north-east England. The population studied was about 2.05 million (UK census 1991) which included 6 adjacent health administrative areas. We have fully described our case-finding methods elsewhere[10]. Briefly these included:

1. A request to all physicians and relevant surgeons in this region for details of all their patients with known PBC.
2. Hospital admission data on Regional Information Systems for all 13 hospitals in the region (ICD-9 code 571.6).
3. Examination of all hospital immunology laboratory data for patients with AMA positive 1 in 40 or greater by indirect immunofluorescence (207 000 autoimmune profiles were examined over 8 years).
4. All listings from the Office of National Statistics (ONS) for ICD-9 code 571.6 anywhere on a death certificate in individuals from the defined geographical area.

Our case definition was as follows:

1. A case was regarded as definitive if all 3 of the following criteria were met:

   a. AMA positive $\geq$ 1 in 40.
   b. Cholestatic LFTs.
   c. Diagnostic or compatible liver histology.

2. A case was regarded as probable if any two of the above three were confirmed (and if AMA and LFTs only, these had to be abnormal on two or more occasions).

Hospital case records were examined on all cases who had attended hospital. Cases who had never attended hospital were traced through their family

Table 2   North-east England PBC epidemiology

Total cases	770
Definite cases	472
Probable cases	298
Incident cases (1987–1994)	468
Definite	239
AMA-negative PBC	13
Normal LFTs, positive AMA, diagnostic biopsy	6
Abnormal LFTs, positive AMA (both ×2 at least)	210
Prevalent cases	
1987	304
1994	514

Table 3   North-east England PBC epidemiology – prevalence in 1994

Whole region	Total population	$251/10^6$
	Adult population	$309/10^6$
	Women over 40 years	$940/10^6$
Within region		
Sunderland	Total population	$152/10^6$
	Women over 40 years	$594/10^6$
North of Tyne	Total population	$396/10^6$
	Women over 40 years	$1500/10^6$

doctor (these were very few). All individuals who had never attended hospital or who had stopped hospital follow-up were offered appointments in the Freeman Hospital PBC clinic.

All cases were flagged with the ONS (for information on cause of death).

Results

These are shown in Tables 2 and 3. The rise in prevalence of PBC from 1965 to 1994, using information from an earlier epidemiological study which we carried out[11], is shown in Figure 2. Clearly, these are by far the highest ever recorded figures for the prevalence of PBC world wide. It will be seen that, among women over age 40, almost one in 750 in the area of North of Tyne have definite or probable PBC. Since there have been interested physicians in North of Tyne for 20 years and since a number of case-finding exercises have been carried out over that period, most recently and thoroughly for the 8 years from 1987 to 1994 inclusive, the remarkable rise in incidence cannot merely be attributed to our increased interest in and knowledge of the disease; we are seeking ways to examine this problem further.

NEW INFORMATION ABOUT THE NATURAL HISTORY OF PBC

From the above study, among the 770 cases, 311 (55.5%) were asymptomatic at the time of presentation (or 'detection'), 249 (44.5%) were symptomatic at presentation. A further 210 were detected as a result of case finding studies.

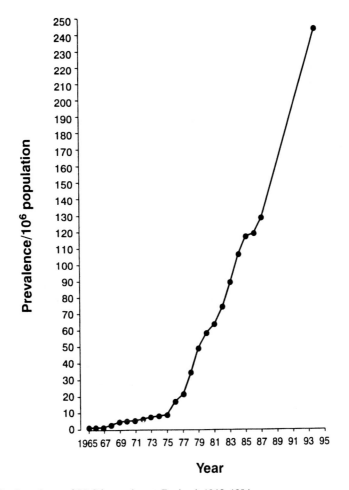

Figure 2   Prevalence of PBC in north-east England, 1965–1994.

The median follow-up among these 770 cases was 6.3 years (range 2.03–29.5). The total mortality was 293 (37.5%) of whom 142 died of causes related to liver disease and 173 either died of liver-related causes or were transplanted. Granted that, earlier in the period, a smaller proportion of individuals were being transplanted, we can now say that, among all patients with PBC in a community, about a quarter will die of liver disease or be transplanted over a follow-up period of 6–8 years.

I would finally suggest that further information which will become available from this cohort may represent the most reliable data available on the natural history of PBC since it is as close as we can come to an unselected group of patients rather than a case series with all its inherent biases, however large the case series may be.

Since this presentation a further study from Swansea (Wales) has indicated prevalence of PBC of $200/10^6$, confirming the upward trend in UK figures[12].

References

1. Mitchison HC, Bassendine MF, Hendrick A, *et al*. Positive antimitochondrial antibody, but normal alkaline phosphatase. Is this primary biliary cirrhosis? Hepatology 1986;6:1279–84.
2. Metcalf JV, Mitchison HC, Palmer JM, Jones DE, Bassendine MF, James OFW. Natural history of early primary biliary cirrhosis. Lancet 1996;348:1399–402.
3. Lindor KD. Early primary biliary cirrhosis: just delayed or different? Hepatology 1997;26:239–40.
4. Long RG, Scheuer PJ, Sherlock S. Presentation and course of asymptomatic primary biliary cirrhosis. Gastroenterology 1977;72:1204–7.
5. Mitchison HC, Lucey MR, Kelly PJ, *et al*. Symptom development and prognosis in primary cirrhosis: a study in two centres. Gastroenterology 1990;99:778–84.
6. Balasubramanian K, Grambsch PM, Wiesner RH, *et al*. Diminished survival in asymptomatic primary biliary cirrhosis: a prospective study. Gastroenterology 1990;98:1567–71.
7. Mahl RC, Shockcor W, Boyer JL. Primary biliary cirrhosis: survival of a large cohort of symptomatic and asymptomatic patients followed for 24 years. J Hepatol 1994;20:707–13.
8. Hamlyn AN, Sherlock S. The epidemiology of primary biliary cirrhosis: a survey of mortality in England and Wales. Gut 1974;15:473–9.
9. Metcalf JV, James OFW. The geoepidemiology of primary biliary cirrhosis. Semin Liver Dis 1997;17:13–22.
10. Metcalf JV, Gray J, Howel D, Bhopal RS, James OFW. Incidence and prevalence of primary biliary cirrhosis in the city of Newcastle upon Tyne, England. Int J Epidemiol 1997;26:830–6.
11. Myszor M, James OFW. The epidemiology of primary biliary cirrhosis in northern England: an increasingly common disease? Q J Med 1990;75:377–85.
12. Kingham JGC, Parker DR. The association between primary biliary cirrhosis and coeliac disease: a study of relative prevalences. Gut 1998;42:120–2.

2
Immune basis for PBC

M. F. BASSENDINE

PBC is characterized by disease-specific, non-organ-specific (antimito-chondrial (AMA) and/or antinuclear (ANA)) autoantibodies and is generally considered to be an autoimmune disorder. In common with other auto-immune diseases, it is thought that inherited factors play a role in determin-ing disease susceptibility. The major evidence in support of this has come from family studies. The risk of PBC is much higher in close relatives of patients with the disease than in the rest of the population[1,2]. The prevalence of PBC in first-degree relatives of patients has been estimated to be as high as 6420/100 000 (6.4%), significantly higher than the highest reported whole-population prevalence[3].

Limited data are available regarding the genetic loci responsible for PBC susceptibility[4]. Most attention has focused on the major histocompatibility complex (MHC) on chromosome 6. An MHC association with the class II allele HLA DR8 has now been demonstrated in several genotyping studies involving different populations[5-7]. Although this association is strong, the risk associated with HLA DR8 only accounts for a minority of cases. An association has also been demonstrated with the presence of a null allele at the C4 locus within the class III MHC region.[8] Other candidate susceptiblity immunogenetic loci have been studied, including a promoter polymorphism at position −308 of the promoter region of the pro-inflammatory cytokine tumor necrosis factor-α (TNF-α) gene[9,10] and *TAP1&2* genes[11].

The development of autoantibodies appears to be a very early serological marker of PBC; AMA can be detected in patients before the development of abnormal liver function tests and long before the onset of symptoms[12,13]. However, a small minority of patients have the clinical, biochemical and histological features of PBC but are AMA negative. Studies of patients with this variant of PBC have shown that antinuclear antibodies (detected by immunofluorescence) are significantly more common than in AMA-positive patients[14,15], leading to the suggestion that this immunologically distinct syndrome be called 'autoimmune cholangitis'. However, as PBC-specific antinuclear antibodies have now been identified, it seems more likely that primary biliary cirrhosis is a syndrome encompassing a spectrum of disorders

Table 1 Mitochondrial and nuclear antigens reacting with PBC-specific autoantibodies

Antigen	% of PBC sera containing reactive autoantibodies
E2 component of pyruvate dehydrogenase complex (PDC)	90–95
E3BP (protein X) component of PDC	90–95
E2 component of 2-oxoglutarate dehydrogenase complex	65–85
E2 component of branched chain oxo-acid dehydrogenase complex	50–55
E1α component of PDC	40–60
E1β component of PDC	<10
Nucleoporin p62	32
Nuclear pore glycoprotein, gp210	10–25
Lamin B receptor	<5
Nuclear dot-associated protein, Sp100	10–30
Promyelocytic leukemia antigen (PML)	10–30

in which the common finding is non-suppurative destructive cholangitis in the presence of any of several serum autoantibodies.

ANTIMITOCHONDRIAL ANTIBODIES

The mitochondrial autoantigens have been identified as components of the 2-oxo acid dehydrogenase multienzyme complexes; pyruvate, 2-oxoglutarate and branched-chain 2-oxo acid dehydrogenase complexes (PDC, OGDC and BCOADC, respectively). These three complexes are among the best-studied examples of multifunctional proteins catalyzing a set of sequential chemical reactions. Each complex occupies a key position in energy metabolism in a cell. PDC links glycolysis to the Krebs cycle, OGDC is in the Krebs cycle itself, and BCOADC is involved in the regulation of the oxidation of the branched-chain amino acids. Each complex consists of multiple copies of at least three enzymes (E1, E2, and E3). In addition, PDC contains a fourth polypeptide, protein X, which plays a structural role as an E3-binding protein and so now has the functional designation E3BP[16]. Mammalian and *Saccharomyces cerevisiae* PDC has a polypeptide chain ratio of $60E1\alpha:60E1\beta:60E2:12E3BP:24E3$[17] and is slightly larger than a ribosome.

The pivotal development in the study of AMA was the cloning of the major 70-kDa mitochondrial antigen[18], which is recognized by antibodies in the sera of more than 90% of patients with PBC. This led to its identification as the E2 component of PDC[19,20], and the demonstration that all sera that reacted with PDC-E2 also reacted with protein X (PDC-E3BP)[19]. It was rapidly shown that AMA often also react with the E2 components of the other two 2-oxo acid dehydrogenase complexes, OGDC[21] and BCOADC[21,22]. The E1α and β components of PDC have also been shown to react with AMA in the sera of a minority of PBC patients (Table 1).

Epitope mapping

The E2 chains of the three 2-oxo acid dehydrogenase complexes are highly segmented structures that have been conserved in evolution: they comprise, from the N terminus, one to three lipoyl domains, a peripheral subunit-binding domain and a large core-forming acyltransferase catalytic domain[23]. Similarly E3BP has a multidomain substructure consisting of an amino-terminal lipoyl domain, followed by an E3-binding domain and then a carboxyl-terminal E2-binding domain[16].

The main immunodominant region (MIR) on PDC-E2 has been mapped to the inner lipoyl domain[24-26]. This prompted several investigations into the exact role of the lipoic acid cofactor (covalently attached to a lysine residue) in autoantibody recognition[20,27]. We have demonstrated that AMA are present at higher titer and react with higher affinity against the lipoylated (vs non-lipoylated) recombinant human inner lipoyl domain[28]. As noted above, autoantibodies reacting with PDC-E2, crossreact with E3BP (protein X) and the MIR on PDC-protein X has also been localized to within its single lipoyl domain[29].

The three-dimensional structure of a lipoyl domain from PDC-E2 of *E. coli* has been determined by means of nuclear magnetic resonance spectroscopy[30,31]. The lipoylation site (lysine residue) is physically exposed at the tip of a tight turn in one of the β-sheets. It would appear, therefore, that AMA in PBC patients' sera recognize this physically exposed lipoylation site and other distinctive surface conformational features at the tip of the β-turn in the lipoyl domain.

Enzyme inhibitory antimitochondrial antibodies

A striking property of AMA in PBC sera is their capacity to rapidly inactivate the catalytic function of the 2-oxo acid dehydrogenase multienzyme complexes *in vitro*[32-34]. This would suggest that the source of the antigenic drive is the intact multienzyme complex rather than a 'mimicking' protein and points to loss of tolerance as the fundamental lesion in PBC. This hypothesis is further supported by a study measuring the functional reactivity of AMA by means of enzyme inhibition against PDC from different sources: mammalian, *Saccharomyces cerevisiae* and *Escherichia coli*. The PBC sera were highly inhibitory of the mammalian PDC (99%), moderately inhibitory for yeast PDC (70%), and weakly inhibitory for *E. coli* PDC (26%)[35].

T-cell responses to pyruvate dehydrogenase complex

Evidence from immunohistochemical studies and fluorescence activated cell sorter analysis of mononuclear cells isolated from PBC liver suggests that the mononuclear cell infiltrate in the portal tracts consists predominantly of activated CD4+ and CD8+ T-lymphocytes and that Th1 cells are the more prominent T-cell subset[36]. Moreover, damage to biliary epithelial cells (BEC) is accompanied by up-regulation of cell-surface markers, such as class II MHC and the adhesion molecule ICAM-1[37] which are typically induced by T-cell cytokines, a finding that suggests local T-cell activation. In view of the expression of class II MHC antigens and adhesion molecules such as ICAM-1, it has been suggested that BEC may be capable of presenting autoantigen to liver-infiltrating CD4+ lymphocytes and of initiating an intrahepatic immune response. We have shown that this is unlikely as human intrahepatic BEC do not express the necessary costimulatory CD28 ligands,

B7-1 or B7-2, at either mRNA or protein levels and are unable to initiate productive T-cell activation characterized by IL-2 production and a lympho-proliferative response *in vitro*[38].

Several studies have been performed looking at T-cell response to the mitochondrial autoantigens[39]. We have shown that peripheral blood T-cell responses to biochemically purified PDC-E2 and E3BP[40,41] are restricted to PBC patients, suggesting a possible role in the disease process. We have also found that the majority of PBC patients responsive to PDC-E2 show a response to both the lipoyl and catalytic domains, suggesting that there are T-cell epitopes throughout the molecule. In contrast, the T-cell cloning experiments of Shimoda *et al.* suggest that, for T-cell clones from 4 PBC patients, there is a single dominant epitope (p163) spanning the lipoyl binding lysine within the lipoyl domain[42]. We have recently shown that the presence or absence of normal lipoylation does not appear to affect the nature of the T-cell response to either the whole lipoyl domain or p163[43]; this is in contrast to the B-cell response.

ANTINUCLEAR ANTIBODIES

Early studies demonstrated that about one third of patients with PBC had 'antinuclear factors'[44]. Two distinct antinuclear antibodies (ANA), one giving a membrane-like pattern of positivity[45] and the other reacting with multiple nuclear dots[46] by immunofluorescence, have subsequently been described and proposed as alternative serological markers in the rare AMA-negative cases. The last decade has seen parallel breakthroughs in this area to those already described for AMA, with the cloning and characterization of a number of nuclear autoantigens, antibodies to which appear to be specifically associated with PBC (Table 1).

ANA against nuclear envelope proteins

Several investigators showed that most of the autoantibodies from patients with PBC that label the nuclear envelope recognize a protein with a molecu-lar mass of about 200 kDa[45,47]. This protein has been identified as the nuclear pore membrane glycoprotein gp210[48]. In one study, 25% of patients were found to have ANA against gp210 and these autoantibodies appeared to be 100% specific for PBC[49].

Another glycoprotein of the nuclear pore complex, p62, has recently also been shown to be an autoantigen in about a third of PBC patients[50] (Table 1). Anti-p62 antibodies are highly specific for PBC but do not colocal-ize with anti-gp210 autoantibodies, so patients positive for one or other ANA appear to represent immunologically distinct subsets. A very small subset of patients with PBC have ANA against an integral protein of the inner nuclear membrane, the lamin B receptor[51].

ANA against 'nuclear dots'

Two nuclear proteins have now been shown to react with ANA against multiple nuclear dots[52]. The first to be cloned was Sp100[53]. This cDNA codes for a protein of unknown function with sequence similarities to several transcriptional transactivating proteins, including HIV-1 nef proteins. A second protein that colocalizes to dot-like nuclear domains, and is aberrantly expressed in promyelocytic leukemia cells (PML) has also been shown to react with ANA in PBC sera[54]. ANA against PML are as highly prevalent and specific for patients with PBC as those against Sp100[54].

At present, it is not clear how these ANA relate to the pathological process of intrahepatic bile duct destruction and/or to possible different etiological factors.

ROLE OF AUTOANTIBODIES IN ETIOPATHOGENESIS?

It has been suggested that the 'syndrome' of PBC is made up of a spectrum of disorders in which the common finding is intrahepatic bile duct destruction in the presence of any of several serum autoantibodies[15]. In AMA-positive cases, the demonstration of target autoantigen (PDC E2 and/or E3BP) or a cross-reactive molecule[55–57] on the plasma membrane of biliary epithelial cells is tantalizing. It may render the cells susceptible to antibody-mediated cytotoxicity. In addition, if the initial T-cell response in PBC is to foreign PDC-E2 and/or PDC-E3BP, and T cells are recruited that react with shared autologous motifs[58], then cytotoxic T-cell responses would be aimed at the BEC with membrane expression of the autoantigen.

Over the last decade, considerable progress has been made in understanding immunological tolerance but the mechanisms of tolerance to antigens expressed exclusively in peripheral organs have not yet been clearly defined. It is to be hoped that the cloning and characterization of the mitochondrial and nuclear antigens to which loss of tolerance occurs in primary biliary cirrhosis will allow antigen-specific immunotherapy to become a realistic possibility within the next decade.

References

1. Bach N, Schaffner F. Familial primary biliary cirrhosis. J Hepatol 1994;20:698–701.
2. Brind AM, Bray GP, Portmann BC, Williams R. Prevalence and pattern of familial disease in primary biliary cirrhosis. Gut 1995;36:615–17.
3. Metcalf JV, Bhopal RS, Gray J, Howel D, James OFW. Incidence and prevalence of primary biliary cirrhosis in the city of Newcastle upon Tyne, England. Int J Epidemiol 1997;26(4):830–6.
4. Gregory WL, Bassendine MF. Genetic factors in primary biliary cirrhosis. J Hepatol 1994;20:689–92.
5. Underhill J, Donaldson P, Bray G, Doherty D, Portmann B, Williams R. Susceptiblity to primary biliary cirrhosis is associated with the HLA-DR8-DQB1*0402 haplotype. Hepatology 1992;16:1404–8.
6. Gregory WL, Mehal W, Dunn AN, et al. Primary biliary cirrhosis: contribution of HLA class II allele DR8. Q J Med 1993;86:393–9.
7. Onishi S, Sakamaki T, Maeda T, et al. DNA typing of HLA class II genes; DRB1*0803 increases the susceptibility of Japanese to primary biliary cirrhosis. J Hepatol 1994;21(6):1053–60.
8. Manns MP, Bremm A, Scheider PM, et al. HLA-DRw8 and complement C4 deficiency as risk factors in primary biliary cirrhosis. Gastroenterology 1991;101:1367–73.
9. Gordon MA, Gleeson D, Oppenheim E, di Giovine FS, Camp NC, Duff GW. Tumour necrosis factor genetic polymorphisms and primary biliary cirrhosis. Hepatology 1996;24:166A.

10. Watt FE, Grove J, Daly AK, Day CP, Bassendine MF, Jones DEJ. Tumour necrosis factor-308 polymorphism and disease progression in primary biliary cirrhosis. Gastroenterology 1997;112:A1414.
11. Gregory WL, Daly AK, Dunn AN, et al. Analysis of HLA-class-II-encoded antigen-processing genes TAP1 and TAP2 in primary biliary cirrhosis. Q J Med 1994;87:237–44.
12. Mitchison HC, Bassendine MF, Hendrick AM, et al. Positive antimitochondrial antibody but normal liver function tests: is this primary biliary cirrhosis? Hepatology 1986;6:1279–84.
13. Metcalf JV, Mitchison HC, Palmer JM, Jones DEJ, Bassendine MF, James OFW. Natural history of early primary biliary cirrhosis. Lancet 1996;348:1399–402.
14. Michieletti P, Wanless IR, Katz A, et al. Antimitochondrial antibody negative primary biliary cirrhosis: a distinct syndrome of autoimmune cholangitis. Gut 1994;35(2):260–5.
15. Lacerda MA, Ludwig J, Dickson ER, Jorgensen RA, Lindor MD. Antimitochondrial antibody-negative primary biliary cirrhosis. Am J Gastroenterol 1995;90(2):247–9.
16. Maeng CY, Yazdi MA, Reed LJ. Stoichiometry of binding of mature and truncated forms of the dihydrolipoamide dehydrogenase-binding protein to the dihydrolipoamide acetyl-transferase core of the pyruvate dehydrogenase complex from Saccharomyces cerevisiae. Biochemistry 1996;35:5879–82.
17. Maeng C-Y, Yazdi MA, Niu X-D, Lee HY, Reed LR. Expression, purification, and charac-terisation of the dihydrolipoamide dehydrogenase-binding protein of the pyruvate dehydro-genase complex from Saccharomyces cerevisiae. Biochemistry 1994;33:13801–7.
18. Gershwin ME, Mackay IR, Sturgess A, Coppel RL. Identification and specificity of a cDNA encoding the 70 kD mitochondrial antigen recognized in primary biliary cirrhosis. J Immunol 1987;138:3525–31.
19. Yeaman SJ, Fussey SP, Danner DJ, James OFW, Bassendine MF. Primary biliary cirrhosis: identification of two major M2 mitochondrial autoantigens. Lancet 1988;1:1067–70.
20. Van de Water J, Gershwin ME, Leung P, Ansari A, Coppel RA. The autoepitope of the 74-kD mitochondrial autoantigen of primary biliary cirrhosis corresponds to the functional site of dihydrolipoamide acetyltransferase. J Exp Med 1988;167:1791–9.
21. Fussey SPM, Guest JR, James OFW, Bassendine MF, Yeaman SJ. Identification and analy-sis of the major M2 autoantigens in primary biliary cirrhosis. Proc Natl Acad Sci USA 1988;85:8654–8.
22. Surh CD, Danner DJ, Ahmed A, et al. Reactivity of primary biliary cirrhosis sera with a human fetal liver cDNA clone of branched-chain a-keto acid dehydrogenase dihydrolipo-amide acyltransferase, the 52 kDa mitochondrial autoantigen. Hepatology 1989;9:63–8.
23. Perham RN. Domains, motifs and linkers in 2-oxo acid dehydrogenase multienzyme com-plexes: a paradigm in the design of a multifunctional protein. Biochemistry 1991;30:8501–12.
24. Fussey SP, Bassendine MF, James OFW, Yeaman SJ. Characterisation of the reactivity of autoantibodies in primary biliary cirrhosis. FEBS Lett 1989;246(1–2):49–53.
25. Fussey SPM, Bassendine MF, James OFW, Yeaman SJ. The lipoate-containing domain of PDC E2 contains the main immunogenic region of the 70 kD M2 autoantigen in primary biliary cirrhosis. Ann NY Acad Sci 1989;573:444–6.
26. Surh CD, Coppel R, Gershwin ME. Structural requirement for autoreactivity on human pyruvate dehydrogenase-E2, the major autoantigen of primary biliary cirrhosis. J Immunol 1990;144:3367–74.
27. Tuaillon N, Andre C, Briand JP, Penner E, Muller S. A lipoyl synthetic octapeptide of dihydrolipoamide acetyltransferase specifically recognised by anti-M2 autoantibodies in primary biliary cirrhosis. J Immunol 1992;148:445–50.
28. Quinn J, Diamond AG, Palmer JM, Bassendine MF, James OFW, Yeaman SJ. Lipoylated and unlipoylated domains of human PDC-E2 as autoantigens in primary biliary cirrhosis: significance of lipoate attachment. Hepatology 1993;18(6):1384–91.
29. Fussey SP, Lindsay JG, Fuller C, et al. Autoantibodies in primary biliary cirrhosis: analysis of reactivity against eukaryotic and prokaryotic 2-oxo acid dehydrogenase complexes. Hepatology 1991;13(3):467–74.
30. Green JD, Laue ED, Perham RN, Ali ST, Guest JR. Three-dimensional structure of a lipoyl domain from the dihydrolipoyl acetyltransferase component of the pyruvate dehydrogenase multienzyme complex of Escherichia coli. J Mol Biol 1995;248:328–43.
31. Dardel F, Davis AL, Laue ED, Perham RN. Three-dimensional structure of the lipoyl domain from Bacillus stearothermophilus pyruvate dehydrogenase complex. J Mol Biol 1993;229:1037–48.

32. Van de Water J, Fregeau D, Davis P, et al. Autoantibodies of primary biliary cirrhosis recognize dihydrolipoamide acetyltransferase and inhibit enzyme function. J Immunol 1988;141:2321–4.
33. Fregeau DR, Davis PA, Danner DJ, et al. Antimitochondrial antibodies of primary biliary cirrhosis recognize dihydrolipoamide acyltransferase and inhibit enzyme function of the branched chain a-ketoacid dehydrogenase complex. J Immunol 1989;142:3815–20.
34. Fregeau DR, Prindiville T, Coppel RL, Kaplan M, Dickinson RE, Gershwin ME. Inhibition of a-ketoglutarate dehydrogenase activity by a distinct population of autoantibodies recognising dehydrolipoamide succinyltransferase in primary biliary cirrhosis. Hepatology 1990;11:975–81.
35. Teoh KL, Mackay IR, Rowley MJ, Fussey SP. Enzyme inhibitory autoantibodies to pyruvate dehydrogenase complex in primary biliary cirrhosis differ for mammalian, yeast and bacterial enzymes: implications for molecular mimicry. Hepatology 1994;19(4):1029–33.
36. Harada K, Van de Water J, Leung PS, et al. In situ nucleic acid hybridization of cytokines in primary biliary cirrhosis: predominance of the Th1 subset. Hepatology 1997;25(4):791–6.
37. Yasoshima M, Nakanuma Y, Van de Water J, Gershwin ME. Immunohistochemical analysis of adhesion molecules in the micro-environment of portal tracts in relation to aberrant expression of PDC-E2 and HLA-DR on the bile ducts in primary biliary cirrhosis. J Pathol 1995;175(3):319–25.
38. Leon MP, Bassendine MF, Wilson JL, Ali S, Thick M, Kirby JA. Immunogenicity of biliary epithelium: Investigation of antigen presentation to CD4+ T cells. Hepatology 1996; 24:561–7.
39. Van de Water J, Ansari A, Prindiville T, et al. Heterogeneity of autoreactive T cell clones specific for the E2 component of the pyruvate dehydrogenase complex in primary biliary cirrhosis. J Exp Med 1995;181(2):723–33.
40. Jones DEJ, Palmer JM, Yeaman SJ, James OFW, Bassendine MF, Diamond AG. T-cell responses to components of pyruvate dehydrogenase complex in primary biliary cirrhosis. Hepatology 1995;21:995–1002.
41. Jones DEJ, Palmer JM, Yeaman SJ, Bassendine MF, Diamond AG. T-cell responses to native human proteins in primary biliary cirrhosis. Clin Exp Immunol 1997;107:562–8.
42. Shimoda S, Nakamura M, Ishibishi H, Hayashida K, Niho Y. HLA DRB4 0101-restricted immunodominant T-cell autoepitope of pyruvate dehydrogenase complex in primary biliary cirrhosis: evidence of molecular mimicry in human autoimmune disease. J Exp Med 1995;181:1835–45.
43. Palmer JM, Jones DEJ, Yeaman SJ, Diamond AG, Bassendine MF. T-cell responses to the putative dominant T-cell autoepitope in primary biliary cirrhosis: the role of lipoylation. Hepatology 1997;26(4):439A.
44. Doniach D, Roitt IM, Walker JG, Sherlock S. Tissue antibodies in primary biliary cirrhosis, active chronic (lupoid) hepatitis, cryptogenic cirrhosis and other liver diseases and their clinical implications. Clin Exp Immunol 1966;1:237–62.
45. Lozano F, Pares A, Borche L, et al. Autoantibodies against nuclear envelope-associated proteins in primary biliary cirrhosis. Hepatology 1988;8:930–8.
46. Powell F, Schoeter AL, Dickson ER. Antinuclear antibodies in primary biliary cirrhosis. Lancet 1984;1:288–9.
47. Lassoued K, Guilly MN, Andre C, et al. Autoantibodies to 200 kD polypeptide(s) of the nuclear envelope: a new serologic marker of primary biliary cirrhosis. Clin Exp Immunol 1988;74(2):283–8.
48. Courvalin J-C, Worman HJ. Nuclear envelope protein autoantibodies in primary biliary cirrhosis. Semin Liver Disease 1997;17:79–90.
49. Lassoued K, Brenard R, Degos F, et al. Antinuclear antibodies directed to a 200-kilodalton polypeptide of the nuclear envelope in primary biliary cirrhosis. A clinical and immunological study of a series of 150 patients with primary biliary cirrhosis. Gastroenterology 1990;99(1):181–6.
50. Wesierska-Gadek J, Honenauer H, Hitchman E, Penner E. Autoantibodies against nucleoporin p62 constitute a novel marker of primary biliary cirrhosis. Gastroenterology 1996; 110:840–7.
51. Courvalin JC, Lassoued K, Worman HJ, Blobel G. Identification and characterisation of autoantibodies against the nuclear envelope lamin B receptor from patients with primary biliary cirrhosis. J Exp Med 1990;172(3):961–7.

52. Szostecki C, Guldner HH, Will H. Autoantibodies against nuclear dots in primary biliary cirrhosis. Semin Liver Dis 1997;17:71–8.
53. Szostecki C, Guldner HH, Netter HJ, Will H. Isolation and characterisation of cDNA encoding a human nuclear antigen predominantly recognised by autoantibodies from patients with primary biliary cirrhosis. J Immunol 1990;145:4338–47.
54. Sternsdorf T, Gulder HH, Szostecki C, Grotzinger T, Will H. Two nuclear dot associated proteins, PML and Sp100, are often co-autoimmunogenic in patients with primary biliary cirrhosis. Scand J Immunol 1995;42(2):257–68.
55. Joplin R, Gordon Lindsay J, Johnson GD, Strain A, Neuberger J. Membrane dihydrolipo-amide acetyltransferase (E2) on human biliary epithelial cells in primary biliary cirrhosis. Lancet 1992;339:93–4.
56. Van de Water J, Turchany J, Leung PS, et al. Molecular mimicry in primary biliary cirrhosis. Evidence for biliary epithelial expression of a molecule cross-reactive with pyruvate dehydrogenase complex-E2. J Clin Invest 1993;91(6):2653–64.
57. Joplin RE, Johnson GD, Matthews JB, et al. Distribution of pyruvate dehydrogenase dihydrolipoamide acetyltransferase (PDC-E2) and another mitochondrial marker in salivary gland and biliary epithelium from patients with primary biliary cirrhosis. Hepatology 1994;19:1375–80.
58. Mamula MJ, Lin RH, Janeway CA, Hardin JA. Breaking T cell tolerance with foreign and self co-immunogens: a study of autoimmune T and B cell epitopes of cytochrome c. J Immunol 1992;149:789–95.

3
Isolation and cloning of antimitochondrial antibodies

R. JOPLIN

Primary biliary cirrhosis (PBC) is characterized by the presence of M2 antimitochondrial antibodies (AMA) in a patient's serum. These antibodies react with components of the oxo-acid dehydrogenase mitochondrial multi-enzyme complexes. The part played by these AMA in damage to bile ducts in PBC is not known but the antibodies are present before any abnormality is detectable, either in liver function or histology. Thus, detection of AMA is considered a reliable early marker for PBC[1]. Although M2 AMA have been extensively characterized with respect to their reaction with components of the oxo-acid dehydrogenase complexes, the important target antigens in the liver of patients with PBC remain undetermined. Identification of these liver antigens could be important in understanding mechanisms of pathogenesis and/or progression of PBC and purified and cloned AMA are proving useful in identifying these antigens.

Five mitochondrial antigens recognized by M2 AMA have been identified. These antigens are all components of the three related multienzyme complexes, pyruvate dehydrogenase complex (PDC), 2-oxoglutarate dehydrogenase complex (OGDC) and branched chain oxo-acid dehydrogenase complex (BCOADC)[2]. Each complex is composed of multiple copies of several different enzymes, termed E1, E2 and E3, and PDC contains an additional component termed component X (E3-binding protein)[3]. In the case of OGDC and BCOADC, AMA recognize a single protein in each complex; the E2 component. However, when antibodies to PDC are present (in greater than 90% of patients with PBC), they recognize at least two different components of PDC; E2 and component X. In addition, antibodies to PDC-E1 may also be present. Resolution of the M2 mitochondrial antigens by polyacrylamide gel electrophoresis and immunoblotting with serum pooled from several patients with PBC, demonstrates that the five antigens have molecular weights estimated at 68–74 kDa (PDC-E2), 52–56 kDa (BCOADC-E2), 51–52 kDa (PDC-X), 43–48 kDa (OGDC-E2), 30–33 kDa (PDC-E1). Antibody reactivity with several different proteins on immunoblots could result either from antibodies recognizing intrinsically different epitopes which are restricted to the different antigens or multiple bands could equally result from the presence of a single cross-reactive epitope shared by the different molecules. The important issue of whether multiple epitopes or a single cross-reactive epitope is present on the five antigens has to a large extent been resolved. More than 90% of patients have antibodies to PDC-E2 and X but only 50% of patients have AMA that recognize all three oxo-acid dehydrogenase complexes, suggesting that epitopes in BCOADC and OGDC are independent of the epitopes in PDC-E2[4]. This suggestion is further supported by biochemical and epitope mapping studies. In addition, purified AMA and monoclonal antibody techniques are enabling more detailed studies into the fine specificity of antibodies produced by individual lymphocyte clones.

AMA can be generated in a number of different ways. They can be isolated from patients by techniques such as affinity purification from patients' serum[5] or monoclonal antibodies can be raised from the patient's lymphocytes[6-8]. Human monoclonal antibodies have now been raised from the peripheral blood of patients with PBC in a number of laboratories around the world, and clones which produce antibodies specific for PDC[7,8] and OGDC[6] have been generated. In addition, combinatorial antibodies have been raised from the lymph nodes of patients with PBC[9]. The reaction of these human monoclonal and combinatorial antibodies to PDC-E2 and OGDC-E2 has been found to be mutually exclusive; antibodies that react with PDC-E2 do not crossreact with OGDC-E2 and *vice versa*. These data support the concept that individual discrete epitopes are present in the different OGDC-E2 and PDC-E2 components, confirming previous epitope mapping studies. However, although some monoclonal antibodies to PDC-E2 react only with E2, others react with both E2 and X suggesting the possibility of a genuine crossreactive epitope shared by both E2 and X components of PDC. Considerable structural and functional homology exists between PDC-E2 and PDC-X and antibodies that recognize the immunodominant lipoyl domains of PDC-E2 frequently also react with the single lipoyl domain of component X[4].

Another approach to generating AMA is to artificially raise polyclonal or monoclonal antibodies by immunization of animals either with mitochondria or specific antigen. Polyclonal antibodies to PDC-E2 and PDC-X have been generated by immunizing rabbits with gel purified bovine antigen[4,10] while monoclonal antibodies to PDC-E2 have been raised by immunizing mice either with mitochondria or recombinant human PDC-E2[11,12]. Although these antibodies have been produced artificially and are not the naturally occurring antibodies involved in PBC, they have been useful in studying the distribution and nature of antigens recognized by AMA in the liver of patients with PBC. The mitochondrial multienzyme complexes recognized by AMA are ubiquitously present in all aerobic cells. Thus, any role in the highly localized damage to biliary ducts in PBC is difficult to explain. However, although liver is known to contain the mitochondrial antigens recognized by AMA, there may also be other antigens in liver with which AMA react.

A number of studies have now shown that polyclonal anti-PDC-E2 and some monoclonal antibodies to PDC-E2 react differently with the biliary epithelium of patients with PBC than controls. By immunohistochemistry of normal liver, all antibodies to PDC-E2 show a characteristic pattern of particulate mitochondrial staining on all cell types in the section. In PBC liver, however, the epithelial lining of a proportion of bile ducts shows very high intensity of an antigen which appears concentrated at the lumenal pole of the biliary epithelial cells, specifically in patients with PBC[12,13]. The staining is diffuse and appears not to be restricted to mitochondria. This striking abnormal distribution of antigen recognized by anti-PDC-E2 has also been observed on biliary epithelium in biopsy samples from patients with early PBC (stage I/II)[14], suggesting that altered distribution of this antigen may be one of the earliest events in the liver of patients with PBC. Furthermore, biliary epithelium in the allografts of patients who had undergone orthotopic liver transplantation for PBC, also showed the atypical distribution of antigen recognized by some, but not all, antibodies to PDC-E2[15,16]. Finally, some PDC-E2-specific combinatorial antibodies raised from the portal lymph nodes of patients with PBC also showed the atypical distribution of binding to biliary epithelium in the liver of patients with PBC[15], suggesting that patients' AMA and not simply antibodies raised in animal models could produce this atypical staining pattern. Thus, it is possible that abnormal expression of a biliary epithelial cell antigen in PBC could be involved in breakdown of tolerance to self antigens and lead to immune recognition and damage to bile ducts.

Previously, we described a method to purify biliary epithelial cells (BEC) from the livers of patients with PBC and controls[17]. We have used these purified BEC to investigate the nature of BEC antigens recognized by AMA. Studies were undertaken to localize antibody binding to specific subcellular structures of purified BEC. In controls (BEC from normal liver and other cholestatic conditions), polyclonal rabbit anti-PDC-E2 showed a simple mitochondrial distribution, but, in BEC from patients with PBC, staining was more intense and diffuse. Using special staining techniques, antigen was found to be associated not only with mitochondria, but also with the external aspect of the plasma membrane of BEC isolated from patients with PBC but not controls. Identical results were obtained whether rabbit polyclonal anti-PDC-E2 or human anti-PDC which had been affinity purified from the serum of patients with PBC was used[18]. Furthermore, Gershwin and co-workers demonstrated that mouse monoclonal anti-PDC-E2 also reacted with the plasma membrane of BEC in histological sections of liver of patients with PBC[19].

The identity of the abnormally distributed antigen in BEC in PBC is unknown but several possibilities exist, such as defects in PDC-E2 degradation or targeting pathways. However, compelling evidence now exists to suggest that the high intensity antigen is not PDC-E2 but a different antigen with a crossreactive epitope. On sections of PBC liver, some monoclonal and combinatorial antibodies to PDC-E2 show a simple, particulate mitochondrial distribution on BEC. However, other antibodies (polyclonal anti-PDC-E2[13] and some human and murine monoclonal antibodies to PDC-

E2[12,15]) exhibit the high intensity of binding to BEC in patients with PBC. Thus, not all monoclonal antibodies that react with PDC-E2, react with BEC in the same way. These observations provide strong circumstantial evidence to support the concept that biliary epithelial cells contain a different antigen which has an epitope crossreactive with an epitope of PDC-E2.

We have investigated the nature of the BEC antigens in PBC by Western blotting studies using BEC purified from the liver of patients with PBC and controls and AMA affinity purified from the serum of patients with PBC[20]. However, these experiments have failed to demonstrate any non-PDC antigen recognized by AMA in BEC. Analysis of total biliary epithelial cellular protein revealed reaction of affinity purified AMA with two major antigens with approximate molecular weights of 70 kDa and 50 kDa which migrated with E2 and X components of purified human heart PDC. Minor reaction with a protein of approximately 30 kDa was also observed (PDC-E1). No difference was observed between the E2 components in PBC and controls. However, higher density of the 50-kDa protein was noted in BEC prepared from the liver of patients with PBC relative to BEC prepared from controls. Furthermore, in subcellular fractionation studies, the 50-kDa antigen was detected in the plasma membrane fraction, while E2 appeared only in the fraction containing mitochondria. Thus, the data support the concept that the plasma membrane antigen recognized by anti-PDC-E2/X in the biliary epithelium of patients with PBC may be PDC-X or another crossreactive antigen. Further studies are required to investigate these possibilities more fully. The availability of new monoclonal reagents will help in elucidation of the nature of biliary epithelial cell antigens in PBC and their role in immunological recognition and damage to bile ducts.

References

1. Mitchison HC, Bassendine MF, Hendrick A, et al. Positive antimitochondrial antibody but normal liver function tests: is this primary biliary cirrhosis? Hepatology 1986;6:1279–84.
2. Yeaman SJ. The 2-oxo-acid dehydrogenase complexes: recent advances. Biochem J 1989;257:625–32.
3. De Marucci J, Lindsay JG. Component X – an immunologically distinct polypeptide associated with mammalian pyruvate dehydrogenase multienzyme complex. Eur J Biochem 1985;149:641–8.
4. Bassendine MF, Fussey SPM, Mutimer DJ, et al. Identification and characterization of four M2 mitochondrial autoantigens in primary biliary cirrhosis. Semin Liver Dis 1989;9:124–31.
5. Palmer JM, Bassendine MF, James OJ, et al. Human pyruvate dehydrogenase complex as an autoantigen in primary biliary cirrhosis. Clin Sci 1993;85:289–93.
6. Fukushima N, Nakamura M, Matsui M, et al. Establishment and structural analysis of human M2 component of the 2-oxoglutarate dehydrogenase complex from a patient with primary biliary cirrhosis. Int Immunol 1995;7:1047–55.
7. Leung PSC, Krams S, Munoz S, et al. Characterization and epitope mapping of human monoclonal antibodies to PDC-E2, the immunodominant autoantigen in primary biliary cirrhosis. J Autoimmun 1992;5:703–18.
8. Thomson RK, Davis Z, Palmer JM, et al. Functional and immunogenetic analysis of anti-PDC specific monoclonal antibodies derived from a patient with PBC. J Hepatol 1997;26:113A.
9. Cha S, Leung PSC, Gershwin ME, et al. Use of a combinatorial immunoglobulin library to generate antibodies to pyruvate dehydrogenase complex (PDC-E2), the major autoantigen of primary biliary cirrhosis. Proc Natl Acad Sci USA 1993;90:2527–31.

10. Hunter A, Lindsay JG. Immunology and biosynthesis of the 2 oxoglutarate dehydrogenase multienzyme complex. Eur J Biochem 1986;155:103–9 E2.
11. Bjorkland A, Mendel Hartvig I, Nelson BD, et al. Primary biliary cirrhosis (PBC) – characterization of a monoclonal antibody (PBC-moab) having specificity identical with disease associated autoantibodies. Scand J Immunol 1991;33:749–53.
12. Van de Water J, Ansari AA, Surh CD, et al. Evidence for the targeting by 2-oxo-dehydrogenase enzymes in the T cell response of primary biliary cirrhosis. J Immunol 1991;146:89–94.
13. Joplin R, Lindsay JG, Hubscher SG, et al. Distribution of dihydrolipoamide acetyltransferase (E2) in the liver and portal lymph nodes of patients with primary biliary cirrhosis: an immunohistochemical study. Hepatology 1991;14:442–7.
14. Tsuneyama K, Van de Water J, Leung PSC, et al. Abnormal expression of PDC-E2 on the luminal surface of biliary epithelium occurs before MHC Class II and BB1/B7 expression. Hepatology 1995;21:1031–7.
15. Van de Water J, Turchany J, Leung PSC, et al. Molecular mimicry in primary biliary cirrhosis. Evidence for biliary epithelial expression of a molecule cross-reactive with pyruvate dehydrogenase complex-E2. J Clin Invest 1993;91:2653–64.
16. Neuberger JMN, Wallace LL, Joplin R, et al. Hepatic distribution of E2 component of pyruvate dehydrogenase complex after transplantation. Hepatology 1995;22:798–801.
17. Joplin R, Strain AJ, Neuberger JMN. Biliary epithelial cells from the liver of patients with primary biliary cirrhosis: isolation, characterization and short-term culture. J Pathol 1990;162:255–60.
18. Joplin R, Wallace LL, Johnson GD, et al. Subcellular localization of pyruvate dehydrogenase dihydrolipoamide acetyltransferase in human intrahepatic biliary epithelial cells. J Pathol 1995;176:381–90.
19. Nakanuma Y, Tsuneyama K, Kono N, et al. Biliary epithelial expression of the pyruvate dehydrogenase complex in primary biliary cirrhosis: an immunohistochemical and immunoelectron microscopic study. Hum Pathol 1995;26:92–8.
20. Joplin R, Wallace LL, Lindsay JG, et al. The human biliary epithelial cell plasma membrane antigen in primary biliary cirrhosis: pyruvate dehydrogenase X? Gastroenterology 1997;113:1727–33.

4
Significance of antimitochondrial antibody profiles in primary biliary cirrhosis

R. KLEIN AND P. A. BERG

INTRODUCTION

As is now well established, PBC can manifest itself as a benign or a progressive disease[1-3]. Several investigators tried to evaluate various clinical and biochemical criteria in order to distinguish these two forms and to predict the clinical outcome; several prognostic models have been established[4-6]. However, although these parameters do seem to allow the determination of the appropriate time for liver transplantation, they are not suitable for differentiating between patients with a benign and those with a progressive course during the early stages of the disease.

From recent retrospective studies, we have evidence that the presence of defined antimitochondrial antibody subtypes correlates with disease activity. Four different antimitochondrial antibody (AMA) types have been described in PBC[7]: anti-M2, -M4, -M8 and -M9. In particular, the presence of complement fixing antibodies to the outer mitochondrial membrane antigens, M4 and M8, is associated with an active or progressive course while patients who are only anti-M2/M9 positive remain in the early stages for a period extending over our observation period of about 18–20 years. Four AMA profiles (A–D) have been defined according to different constellations of these AMA subtypes[3] and were evaluated with respect to their prognostic relevance in different groups of patients[3,8-10]. This seemed to us a logical approach in view of the fact that the association of different AMA subtypes may reflect heightened B-cell and, therefore, increased immunological activity. In this chapter, we will review the clinical/prognostic relevance of these AMA profiles based on retro- and prospective studies.

CHARACTERIZATION OF MITOCHONDRIAL ANTIGEN SYSTEMS IN PBC AND DEFINITION OF AMA PROFILES

The major characteristics of the four mitochondrial antigen systems in PBC are given in Table 1 and have been recently reviewed in detail[7].

Table 1 Definition and characterization of mitochondrial antigen/antibody systems in PBC

AMA subtypes	Corresponding antigen
anti-M2	Subunits of the 2-oxoacid dehydrogenase complex of the inner mitochondrial membrane, trypsin sensitive
anti-M4	Outer mitochondrial membrane antigen, copurifies with sulfite oxidase, trypsin insensitive
anti-M8	Outer mitochondrial membrane antigen, yet undefined, trypsin sensitive
anti-M9	98-kDa and 59-kDa proteins of a 100 000g supernatant from rat liver mitochondria, associated with glycogen phosphorylase

Table 2 Methods for the detection of AMA subtypes

	Antigens used for the demonstration of AMA by:	
AMA subtypes	ELISA/Western blotting	Complement fixation test
anti-M2	M2-fraction prepared by chloroform release of beef heart mitochondria, pyruvate dehydrogenase from pig heart	Sucrose density 1.24–1.28 from beef heart mitochondria
anti-M4	Sulfite oxidase from chicken liver, ion exchange chromatographically purified fraction from a 100 000g supernatant from rat liver mitochondria*	Purified outer mitochondrial membranes from rat liver, sucrose density gradient 1.08–1.10 from rat liver mitochondria
anti-M8	Chromatographically purified fraction from pig kidney microsomes*	Sucrose density gradient 1.16–1.18 from pig kidney microsomes
anti-M9	Purified fraction obtained by ion exchange chromatography from rat liver mitochondria	Not detectable

* Not detectable by Western blotting.

Anti-M2 antibodies have been primarily detected using an antigen fraction prepared by chloroform treatment of beef heart mitochondria which was shown to contain the enzyme H^+-ATPase. A reaction of the PBC-related AMA with this enzyme could be, however, excluded[11]. Using this so-called M2-fraction in solid-phase assays, about 95% of PBC patients were anti-M2 positive but none of the patients with other hepatic and non-hepatic disorders[12].

Applying the M2-fraction to Western blotting, up to five determinants could be visualized with anti-M2 positive PBC sera[13] which have been identified as subunits of the 2-oxoacid–dehydrogenase complex[14–16]. Most PBC sera react with a 70-kDa protein which corresponds to the E2 subunit of the pyruvate dehydrogenase complex (PDC).

For complement fixation test (CFT), either the M2 fraction or sucrose-density gradients from beef heart mitochondria (gradients 1.24–1.28) can be used, while the PDC is not suitable for this method (Table 2).

Table 3 Definition of AMA profiles and incidence in a large series of 3000 PBC patients

AMA profiles	Antibody constellations	Incidence in 3000 patients: number (%)
A	Only anti-M9 positive (ELISA and Western blot)	100 (3)
B	Only anti-M2 positive (ELISA)	814 (27)
C	Anti-M2/-M4/-M8 positive (ELISA)	1520 (51)
D	Anti-M2/-M4/-M8 positive (ELISA and complement fixation test)	566 (19)

Anti-M4 antibodies react with a trypsin-insensitive antigen of the outer mitochondrial membrane. They can be detected by ELISA or CFT but not by Western blotting[7].

Since anti-M4 antibodies have been shown to react with an enzyme fraction containing sulfite oxidase which proved to be another reliable antigen source for the demonstration of anti-M4 by ELISA, we have applied this preparation in routine tests since 1990[17]. Although other authors were unable to detect anti-M4 using sulfite oxidase[18,19], our findings were confirmed by several laboratories in Germany as well as in Great Britain[20] and Australia (Professor Ian Mackay, personal communication).

For the demonstration of anti-M4 by CFT, however, sulfite oxidase is not suitable, and either purified outer mitochondrial membranes or sucrose-density gradients from rat liver mitochondria (gradients 1.08–1.10) have to be applied (Table 2).

Anti-M8 antibodies also react with an outer membrane antigen which is, however, in contrast to M4, trypsin sensitive and can be prepared especially from pig kidney (Table 2). Like anti-M4, anti-M8 antibodies cannot be visualized by Western blotting[7].

Anti-M9 antibodies were detected by testing anti-M2-positive PBC sera against submitochondrial particles (SMP) from rat liver which are completely devoid of M2. Thus, some of these sera still reacted with these SMP, and the antigen still present on the membranes was named M9. It was further purified by ion exchange chromatography, and this antigen fraction was suitable also for Western blotting (Table 2). Two determinants at 98 and 59 kDa could be visualized. This method turned out to be the only reliable test for anti-M9[21].

Although further studies indicated that M9 is an epitope of glycogen phosphorylase, this commercially available enzyme is not suitable for the demonstration of anti-M9 by ELISA or Western blotting[22].

Anti-M9 antibodies can be detected by ELISA and Western blotting but not by CFT.

From our experience, gained over the past 15 years in AMA subtyping of PBC patients, we can now draw the following conclusions:

1. Anti-M4 and anti-M8 antibodies are always associated with anti-M2 and, like anti-M2, do not occur in any other disease.
2. Anti-M9 antibodies can occur without anti-M2 (rare event, see also Table 3).

Table 4 Biochemical parameters in 100 patients who were anti-M9 positive only (profile A) compared with 2900 patients with classical anti-M2-positive PBC

Biochemical parameters	Anti-M9 positive only (n = 100)	Anti-M2 positive (n = 2900)
AP (IU/L)	456 ± 344	568 ± 423
γ-GT (IU/L)	182 ± 152	233 ± 226
ALAT (IU/L)	51 ± 50	52 ± 66
Bilirubin (mg%)	1.3 ± 2.5	2.3 ± 4.5
IgM (mg%)	374 ± 195	473 ± 324

All figures are mean ± SD.

3. AMA-subtypes are present in the early stages and do not change during the course of PBC in untreated patients or patients treated with UDCA. However, anti-M4/-M8 can disappear during immunosuppressive therapy.
4. For the further evaluation of prognosis, the determination of anti-M2 and anti-M4 by ELISA (and CFT) is sufficient (profile B: anti-M2 versus profile C/D anti-M2 + anti-M4) (see below).
5. Overlap syndromes with other liver disorders have to be excluded.

The definition of the four AMA profiles which resulted from the different antibody constellations as well as their incidence in a large series of 3000 PBC patients is given in Table 3. The comparison of biochemical and histological parameters in the 100 patients with profile A with that of the 2900 patients who were anti-M2 positive (with or without anti-M4/M8) confirmed our previous observation[23] that these only anti-M9-positive patients have the typical constellation of PBC although levels of biochemical parameters are lower than in anti-M2-positive patients (Table 4). Also histology revealed in most instances typical features of PBC but there were only mild inflammatory processes indicating that patients with profile A suffer from a mild form of PBC. However, due to the rare incidence of these patients there seems to be no need for routine testing for anti-M9.

PROGNOSTIC RELEVANCE OF AMA PROFILES

Analysis of AMA profiles in a retrospective study on PBC patients in stage I/II as well as in patients selected for liver transplantation

In a retrospective study of 76 patients who were in stage I/II at the time of first diagnosis and who could be followed for 6–18 years (mean 10 years), it could be shown that 71% of the 44 patients with the profile C/D progressed to stage III/IV (Table 5); nine of them died or required liver transplantation. In contrast, only one of the 32 patients with profile A/B developed histological features of liver cirrhosis[3].

Furthermore, we analyzed sera from patients selected for liver transplantation from different transplantation centers (Table 6). Seventy-four of the 80 patients (93%) had the profile C/D. Interestingly, the remaining six

Table 5 Retrospective analysis of the prognostic relevance of AMA profiles in 76 patients who were in stage I/II at entry into the study

Profile	n	Percentage who had progressed to stage III/IV after 6–18 years
A/B	32	3
C/D	44	71

Table 6 High frequency of the prognostic unfavorable AMA profiles C/D in late-stage PBC patients who had been selected for liver transplantation in three different centers

AMA profile	Number positive		
	Groningen (n = 28)	Tübingen (n = 15)	Berlin (n = 37)
A/B	2*	2*	2*
C/D	26	13	35

*Patients had either an overlap with autoimmune hepatitis or antibodies to nuclear dots (anti-sp100).

patients with profile B all had evidence either for an association with autoimmune hepatitis or they were positive for PBC-specific antinuclear antibodies (antibodies to nuclear dots, anti-sp100) which, at least in our experience, are also indicative of heightened disease activity.

Analysis of AMA profiles in a prospective study based on 200 PBC patients followed for 10 years

In order to substantiate the prognostic relevance of AMA profiles we performed a prospective study in 200 PBC patients in whom AMA profiles had been determined in 1984[10]. All patients were not taking any therapy at this time point. As major criteria for an unfavorable course we defined the necessity for OLT or death due to liver failure, but we also investigated histological progression and increase of bilirubin levels during the course of the disease.

At the beginning of the study, 177 of the 200 patients were in stage I/II of the disease; 23 patients were in stage III/IV. All of the latter patients had the profile C/D; of the stage I/II patients, 102 expressed C/D profile and 75 the A/B profile.

Twelve of the 177 patients with PBC stage I/II died because of their liver disease or had to be transplanted. All of them had the profile C/D (Table 7). Interestingly, at entry into the study, biochemical parameters including AP, transaminases and bilirubin levels, did not differ in these 12 patients from those of 75 patients with profile A/B remaining in stage I/II while IgG and IgM levels were significantly higher in the former group, again underlining the increased immunological activity (Table 8). Furthermore, an increase of bilirubin levels was observed in 42 patients, 41 of whom had the profile C/D (Table 7).

Table 7 Evaluation of the prognostic relevance of AMA profiles in a prospective study of 177 patients in stage I/II at entry into the study followed for a period of up to 10 years

	AMA profiles	
Criteria for progression	A/B (n = 75)	C/D (n = 102)
Necessity for OLT	0	7
Lethal outcome	0	5
Increase of bilirubin (> 1.5 mg%)	1	41

Figures are numbers of patients.

Table 8 Biochemical parameters in 12 patients with profile C/D in stage I/II at entry into the study developing a final stage during the observation period compared with parameters in 75 patients with profile A/B remaining in stage I/II

	Patient profile	
Biochemical parameters	C/D progressing to final stages (n = 12)	A/B remaining in stage I/II (n = 75)
AP (IU)	810 ± 450	419 ± 275
γ-GT (IU)	$262 \pm 122*$	173 ± 130
ALAT (IU)	62 ± 51	45 ± 29
Bilirubin (mg%)	0.8 ± 0.4	0.7 ± 0.4
IgG (mg%)	$1736 \pm 550**$	1299 ± 353
IgM (mg%)	$534 \pm 73**$	359 ± 145

All figures are mean $\pm$ SD. Significantly increased as compared to patients with profile A/B: $*p < 0.05$; $**p < 0.01$.

Table 9 Correlation of histological criteria of progression with the two principal AMA profiles in patients in stage I/II at entry into the study: prospective study for up to 10 years*

AMA profile	n	Percentage progressing to stage III/IV
A/B	58	2
C/D	86	50

*Analysis of 144 patients in stage I/II at entry into the study in whom last biopsy had been performed at least 1–2 years prior to the end of the study.

For the analysis of histological criteria, we included only patients with stage I/II in whom the last liver biopsy had been performed at least 1–2 years prior to the end of the study (n = 144). Half of the patients with profile C/D but only 2% of those with the profile A/B showed a progression to stage III/IV during the observation period (Table 9).

Survival time decreased more rapidly in patients with profile C/D than in patients with profile A/B (Figure 1). From this analysis, it also became evident that observation periods of 6–8 years after first diagnosis in stage I/II seem to be necessary before progression can be documented clinically. Similar observations were made by Mahl et al.[24] who found a median predicted survival from the time of diagnosis of 7.5 years for symptomatic

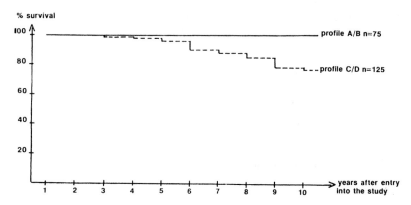

Figure 1 Survival time in 200 patients with PBC followed for up to 10 years in relation to the four AMA profiles. In patients with profile C/D, a decrease in survival time seems to begin 6 years after first presentation.

patients and 16 years for asymptomatic patients. Nyberg and Loof[25] noted diminished survival in their cohort of asymptomatic patients after only 12 years of follow-up. A clear differentiation between the two major courses of PBC may, therefore, become evident only 6 years or even later after first diagnosis in stage I/II, suggesting that shorter observation periods may not be sufficient to estimate the natural course or the efficacy of different therapeutic regimes. Poupon et al. stated that patients with mild disease do not progress to end-stage disease within 4 years[26].

Effect of UDCA therapy on the outcome of PBC in patients with profile C/D in stage I/II at the time of diagnosis

It was not the aim of this prospective study to investigate the effects of different therapeutic regimens on the course of the disease; therefore, it was not a randomized double-blind controlled study. None of the patients received any therapy at entry into the study. However, some patients were treated with UDCA during the follow up, and, from these data, some preliminary conclusions can be drawn.

Thirty-two patients with profile C/D and stage I/II at entry into the study did not receive any therapy during the whole observation period, while, in 45 patients, UDCA was given (mean period of treatment 5 years). Interestingly, death or OLT occurred less frequently in the UDCA-treated group while the histological progression to stage III/IV was only slightly reduced. Also, the increase of bilirubin was not as pronounced as that in the untreated patients (Table 10).

CONCLUDING REMARKS

From these retro- and prospective studies, it emerges that the determination of AMA profiles allows the differentiation between a benign and a more progressive course already at early stages.

Table 10 Influence of UDCA therapy on clinical parameters in PBC stage I/II patients with profile C/D (follow up of 10 years)

Clinical presentation after the end of the observation period	UDCA therapy (n = 45)	No treatment (n = 32)
OLT/death (%)	9	16
Progressed to stage III/IV (%)	36	41
Increased bilirubin		
%	31	53
Increase (mean ± SD)	1.9 ± 2.8*	3.5 ± 6.7

* Significantly lower than in the untreated group ($p < 0.01$).

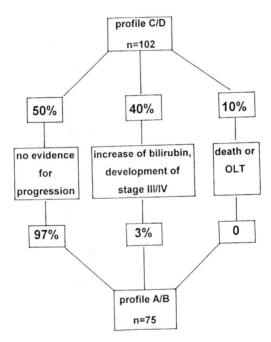

Figure 2 Analysis of the prognostic relevance of AMA profiles in 177 patients with PBC stage I/II in a prospective study (10 years observation period).

Positivity of patients for anti-M4/M8 (profile C/D) who are clinically and histologically still in stage I/II of the disease indicates a heightened risk for a more progressive course. Although, as shown in the prospective study, about 50% of these patients did not progress to late stages within 10 years, the other 50% developed features of liver cirrhosis, and about 10% had died or had to be transplanted within that time (Figure 2). This is in contrast to patients with profile A/B who all remained in early stages during the whole observation period. In a retrospective analysis of 76 stage I/II patients followed for up to 18 years, 71% of 44 patients with profile C/D but only

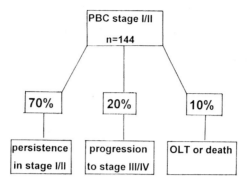

Figure 3 Analysis of the outcome of PBC in 144 patients in stage I/II at first diagnosis in a prospective study (10 years observation period).

3% of 32 profile A/B patients had progressed to late stages; 20% of the profile C/D patients had died or received a liver transplant.

We do not know yet whether patients with profile A/B will ever progress to late stages or progress only very slowly. Some of the patients who presented in 1991 in the retrospective study were, however, followed for more than 20 years and during this prolonged observation period, no progression was observed in the patients with profile A/B. The fact that patients with end-stage PBC selected for liver transplantation hardly ever express the A/B profile is an indirect indicator that patients with profile A/B may suffer only from a mild inflammatory liver process but will not reach the final stages.

These studies also indicate that an observation period of 6–8 years after first diagnosis in stage I/II is necessary before progression can be documented clinically. Thus, according to our observations, a decrease in survival of patients with profile C/D becomes evident about 6 years after the first diagnosis.

Additionally, this prognostic study gave some new insights into the natural course of PBC. Thus, it emerged that about 70% of patients in stage I/II at the time of diagnosis remained in the early stages for the following 10 years while 20% progressed to late stages and a further 10% developed end stage PBC (Figure 3).

The early identification of patients at risk of progression to the advanced stages within 10 years may be, therefore, of relevance also with respect to the mode of therapy, and it could well be that patients with a C/D profile in particular may benefit from a combined therapeutic regimen consisting of UDCA plus either steroids or other immunosuppressive agents.

Acknowledgements

The principal hospitals participating in these studies and kindly providing patients' sera and clinical data were: Wilhelminenspital, Vienna (Prof. Pointner); Medizinische Klinik, University of Essen (Prof. Breuer); Medizinische Klinik I, Kassel (Prof. Pausch); Hartwald Klinik der BfA, Bad

Brückenau (Prof. Zilly); Heinz Kalk-Krankenhaus, Bad Kissingen (Dr. Kalk, Dr. Fischer); Stoffwechselklinik Bad Mergentheim (Prof. Tittor); Medizinische Klinik I, University of Tübingen (Prof. Dölle, Prof. Gregor); DRK-Krankenhaus, Hamburg (Prof. Fintelmann); Department of Pathology, University of Hamburg (Prof. Klöppel); Medizinische Klinik, Esslingen (Prof. Maier); Rudolf Virchow Klinikum, University of Berlin (Prof. Hopf); Division of Hepatology, University of Groningen (Prof. Gips); and several further hospitals and general practitioners in Germany.

This work was supported by the Deutsche Forschungsgemeinschaft, Bonn Bad Godesberg, Be 431/20.

References

1. Roll J, Boyer JL, Barry D, Klatskin G. The prognostic importance of clinical and histologic features in asymptomatic and symptomatic primary biliary cirrhosis. N Engl J Med 1983;308:1–7.
2. Beswick DR, Klatskin G, Boyer JL. Asymptomatic primary biliary cirrhosis. A progress report on long-term follow up and natural history. Gastroenterology 1985;89:267–71.
3. Klein R, Klöppel G, Garbe W, Fintelmann V, Berg PA. Antimitochondrial antibody profiles determined at early stages of primary biliary cirrhosis differentiate between a benign and a progressive course of the disease: A retrospective analysis of 76 patients over 6–18 years. J Hepatol 1991;12:21–7.
4. Dickson ER, Grambsch PM, Fleming TR, et al. Prognosis in primary biliary cirrhosis: Model for decision making. Hepatology 1989;10:1–7.
5. Wiesner RH, Porayko MK, Dickson ER, et al. Selection and timing of liver transplantation in primary biliary cirrhosis and primary sclerosing cholangitis. Hepatology 1992;16:1290–9.
6. Reichen J, Widmer T, Cotting J. Accurate prediction of death by serial determination of galactose elimination capacity in primary biliary cirrhosis: a comparison with the Mayo Model. Hepatology 1991;14:504–10.
7. Berg PA, Klein R. Mitochondrial antigen/antibody systems in primary biliary cirrhosis: revisited. Liver 1995;15:281–92.
8. Klein R, Huizenga JR, Gips CH, Berg PA. Antimitochondrial antibody profiles in patients with primary biliary cirrhosis before orthotopic liver transplantation and titers of AMA-subtypes after transplantation. J Hepatol 1994;20:181–9.
9. Klein R, Berg PA. Prognostische Bedeutung der antimitochondrialen Antikörperprofile A–D bei Patienten mit primär-biliärer Zirrhose. Dtsch Med Wschr 1988;113;1549–53.
10. Klein R, Pointner H, Zilly W, et al. Antimitochondrial antibody profiles in primary biliary cirrhosis distinguish at early stages between a benign and a progressive course: a prospective study on 200 patients followed for 10 years. Liver 1997;17:119–28.
11. Sayers T, Leoutsakos A, Berg PA, Baum H. Antimitochondrial antibodies (AMA) in primary biliary cirrhosis. I. Separation of the PBC antigen activity from mitochondrial ATPase activity. J Bioenerg Biomembr 1981;13:255–67.
12. Berg PA, Klein R, Lindenborn-Fotinos J, Klöppel G. ATPase associated antigen (M2): marker antigen for serological diagnosis of primary biliary cirrhosis. Lancet 1982;2:1423–6.
13. Lindenborn-Fotinos J, Baum H, Berg PA. Mitochondrial antibodies in primary biliary cirrhosis. Further characterization of the M2-antigen by immunoblotting, revealing species and non-species specific determinants. Hepatology 1985;5:763–9.
14. Yeaman SJ, Danner DJ, Mutimer DJ, Fussey SPM, James OFW, Bassendine MF. Primary biliary cirrhosis: identification of two major M2 mitochondrial autoantigens. Lancet 1988;1:1067–70.
15. van de Water J, Surh CD, Leung PSC, et al. Molecular definitions, autoepitopes, and enzymatic activities of the mitochondrial autoantigens of primary biliary cirrhosis. Semin Liver Dis 1989;9:132–7.
16. Bassendine MF, Yeaman SJ. Serological markers of primary biliary cirrhosis: diagnosis, prognosis and subsets. Hepatology 1992;15:545–7.

17. Klein R, Berg PA. Anti-M4 antibodies in primary biliary cirrhosis react with sulfite oxidase, an enzyme of the mitochondrial intermembrane space. Clin Exp Immunol 1991;84:445–8.
18. Davis PA, Leung P, Manns M, *et al.* M4 and M9 antibodies in the overlap syndrome of primary biliary cirrhosis and chronic active hepatitis: epitopes or epiphenomena. Hepatology 1992;16:1128–36.
19. Palmer JM, Yeaman SJ, Bassendine MF, James OFW. M4 and M9 autoantibodies in primary biliary cirrhosis – a negative study. J Hepatol 1993;18:251–4.
20. Bunn CC, McMorrow M. Anti-M4 antibodies measured by a sulphite oxidase ELISA in patients with both anti-centromere and anti-M2 antibodies. Clin Exp Immunol 1995;102:131–6.
21. Klein R, Berg PA. Characterization of a new mitochondrial antigen/antibody system (M9/anti-M9) in patients with anti-M2 positive and anti-M2 negative primary biliary cirrhosis. Clin Exp Immunol 1988;74:68–74.
22. Klein R, Berg PA. Anti-M9 antibodies in sera from patients with primary biliary cirrhosis recognize an epitope of glycogen phosphorylase. Clin Exp Immunol 1990;81:65–71.
23. Klein R, Klöppel G, Fischer R, Fintelmann V, Müting D, Berg PA. The mitochondrial antibody anti-M9 – a marker for the diagnosis of early primary biliary cirrhosis (PBC). J Hepatol 1988;6:299–306.
24. Mahl TC, Shockcor W, Boyer L. Primary biliary cirrhosis: survival of a large cohort of symptomatic and asymptomatic patients followed for 24 years. J Hepatol 1994;20:707–13.
25. Nyberg A, Loof L. Primary biliary cirrhosis: clinical features and outcome, with special reference to asymptomatic disease. Scand J Gastroenterol 1989;24:57–64.
26. Poupon RE, Lindor KD, Cauch-Dudek K, Dickson ER, Poupon R, Heathcote EJ. Combined analysis of randomized controlled trials of ursodeoxycholic acid in primary biliary cirrhosis. Gastroenterology 1997;113:884–90.

5
Chloride/bicarbonate exchange in PBC: a clue for pathogenesis?

J. F. MEDINA AND J. PRIETO

PRIMARY BILIARY CIRRHOSIS: A DISEASE OF UNKNOWN PATHOGENESIS

Primary biliary cirrhosis (PBC), a chronic cholestatic process affecting mainly women, is currently considered to be an autoimmune disease with humoral and cellular immunity directed against mitochondrial antigens or crossreactive epitopes[1,2]. However, the molecular changes which originate the autoimmune reaction and the mechanisms responsible for altered immunoregulation in PBC are unknown. Many questions concerning the pathogenesis of this disease remain to be answered. For example, there are patients with virtually identical disease who do not present antimitochondrial antibodies. Also, there are cases in which antimitochondrial antibodies develop after the initiation of pathological alterations in the liver. It is also intriguing that ursodeoxycholic acid (UDCA), a bile acid which induces bicarbonate-rich choleresis, affords more therapeutic benefit than classical immunosuppressants despite the autoimmune mechanisms involved in the disease[3]. Moreover, there is no explanation for the functional changes and abnormal distribution of cell antigens observed in isolated biliary epithelial cells (BEC) from PBC patients.

A characteristic feature of PBC is its frequent association with the sicca syndrome. Such an association may shed some light when trying to understand pathogenetic aspects of PBC, since it might indicate that the same mechanisms responsible for cholestasis are also involved in the failure of other exocrine glands. The recognized role of anion carriers in the generation of hydroionic fluxes into secretions (e.g. bile and saliva), together with the observed therapeutic effect of a bile acid (UDCA) which stimulates the production of bicarbonate-rich bile, led us to postulate that abnormalities in bicarbonate transport mechanisms might play a role in the pathogenesis of PBC.

ANION EXCHANGERS: PHYSIOLOGICAL ROLE

Sodium-independent Cl^-/HCO_3^- anion exchangers (AE), together with other ion carriers, are important in the regulation of intracellular pH and cell volume[4]. AE participate in the control of intracellular pH acting as acid loaders (or, in other words, as base extruders, HCO_3^- out, Cl^- in) in physiological conditions. AE also have a role in the cell response tending to increase cell volume after shrinkage due to extracellular hypertonic medium. In polarized secretory cells, AE play an essential role in the transport of ions, and secondarily of water, to the lumen. In the liver, it has been shown that both BEC and hepatocytes possess AE activity. It is assumed that AE activity of BEC is considerably superior to that of hepatocytes, since BEC contribute about 24% of total bile flow while accounting for less than 5% of liver cells. It is therefore pertinent to think that any derangement in HCO_3^- secretion mechanisms will have a greater impact on BEC than on hepatocytes.

AE proteins are encoded by a family of genes, three of which (AE1, AE2, and AE3) are now well characterized. AE1 is expressed mainly in erythroid cells and kidney, AE2 is widely expressed in epithelial and mesenchymal tissues, and AE3 is expressed mainly in heart and brain. Several isoforms have been described for the different AE mRNAs and some of them are expressed in a tissue-specific manner.

ANION EXCHANGERS IN THE HEPATOBILIARY TRACT

When we explored the expression of AE genes in the human liver, we found that AE2 but not AE1 is normally expressed in this organ. Transcriptional expression of the AE2 gene was shown by both reverse transcription–polymerase chain reaction (RT–PCR) on liver total RNA[5], and *in-situ* hybridization on slices of liver biopsies[6]. AE2 riboprobes gave hybridization signals in hepatocytes, mainly those in the periportal area (zone 1), as well as in bile ducts, the signal intensity being clearly higher in the latter. In order to analyze the AE2 gene expression at the protein level, we prepared a monoclonal antibody against a 14-mer synthetic peptide derived from the AE2 amino acid sequence. Immunohistochemical studies using this antibody showed specific staining by both indirect immunofluorescence technique on frozen liver sections and immunoperoxidase procedure on formalin-fixed liver[7]. AE2 immunostaining located at the canalicular level in hepatocytes and more intensely at the luminal membrane of small and medium bile ducts. This specific localization of AE2 immunoreactivity is consistent with the postulated role for AE2 protein in the generation of canalicular and ductular bile through bicarbonate secretion.

Interestingly, the apical location of AE2 in bile ducts coincides with the presence at this same location of the cystic fibrosis conductance transmembrane regulator (CFTR). But unlike AE2, which locates apically in both bile ducts and hepatocytes, CFTR is only present in bile ducts. The apical colocalization of CFTR (a cAMP-sensitive Cl^- channel) and AE2 in BEC has suggested a mechanistic model for the secretin-stimulated transport of bicarbonate to the bile and fluidification and alkalinization of canalicular bile. According to this model, the interaction of secretin with its receptor at the basolateral membrane of BEC (a membrane receptor coupled to adenyl cyclase) increases intracellular cAMP concentration, and the subsequent opening of chloride channels at the apical membrane leads to Cl^- efflux. Cl^- efflux and/or intracellular alkalinization (or even CFTR activation by itself) might activate AE2 protein which mediates Cl^-/HCO_3^- exchange, causing Cl^- influx into the cell and HCO_3^- efflux to the lumen. This ion transport system would work in conjunction with a sodium-dependent Cl^-/HCO_3^- exchange at the basolateral membrane (which may provide intracellular HCO_3^-) and with a Na^+/H^+ exchange also present at the basolateral membrane (which may cooperate with AE2 to maintain intracellular pH during the secretory process). The ionic force generated in the lumen will attract water which will pass through water channels present in both basolateral and apical membranes (reviewed in Reference 8).

ANION EXCHANGERS: A ROLE IN THE PATHOGENESIS OF PBC?

With the above information in mind, we have proposed that disturbed AE function can play a role in the pathogenesis of PBC. According to this hypothesis, impaired AE2 gene expression in BEC might reduce the formation of ductular bile contributing to cholestasis, and might also alter intracellular pH regulation leading to functional and antigenic changes in these cells. On the other hand, AE2 dysfunction might also occur in other cell types. In exocrine glands, impaired AE2 might reduce hydroionic fluxes into secretions and thus the formation of saliva and tears, leading to sicca syndrome. In lymphocytes, disturbed anion exchange might alter immunoregulatory activities. And finally, altered AE2 function may affect acid–base transport in osteoclasts and contribute to the hepatic osteodystrophy which is common in PBC.

To investigate whether there was any abnormality in the expression of AE genes in PBC, we first analyzed the levels of AE2 mRNA in the liver in patients with normal liver, in patients with PBC, and in other forms of cirrhosis and cholestasis, using a quantitative PCR procedure[5]. PBC patients were found to have a significant reduction in AE2 mRNA levels as compared with normal livers and with other forms of cirrhosis and cholestasis. When a few cases from UDCA-treated PBC patients were analyzed, the levels of AE2 mRNA in the liver were intermediate between those observed in untreated PBC and controls. A striking significant inverse correlation was found in PBC patients between AE2 mRNA values in the liver and the serum levels of γ-glutamyl transpeptidase, suggesting that reduced AE2 expression might be related to the cholestatic disorder in PBC individuals.

By indirect immunoperoxidase, we analyzed the expression of the AE2 gene at the protein level in formalin-fixed liver specimens from similar groups of patients as for AE2 mRNA analysis[9]. Again, a decrease of AE2 expression was observed in PBC. Immunoreactivity scoring of the different liver structures, i.e. canaliculi, terminal ducts, and interlobular ducts, showed a significant reduction of AE2 immunoreactivity in all three structures in PBC, compared with normal livers and cirrhotic or cholestatic control livers (including a few cases with primary sclerosing cholangitis). In PBC patients receiving UDCA, immunoreactivity scores tended to increase slightly compared with untreated PBC cases, and dichotomous (presence/absence traces) comparison of terminal duct immunoreactivities could discriminate between untreated and UDCA-treated PBC.

Interestingly, we also observed that AE2 immunoreactivity in salivary glands (where AE2 is located mainly in striated duct epithelial cells at the basolateral membrane) is reduced in PBC patients with sicca syndrome (as well as in patients with Sjögren's syndrome unrelated to PBC), while a strong AE2 immunostaining was detected in normal salivary gland[10]. This finding suggests that reduced AE2 expression might be implicated in the pluriglandular exocrine failure accompanying PBC.

Moreover, we found that peripheral blood mononuclear cells (PBMC) from PBC patients manifested abnormalities in the expression of AE genes[5]. Low levels of AE2 transcripts were detected by a quantitative PCR procedure in PBMC from PBC subjects, as compared with healthy subjects and with patients with other forms of cirrhosis or cholestatic disorders. Unlike liver cells, lymphoid cells showed expression of the AE1 gene in addition to the AE2 gene. In PBC individuals, the levels of AE1 mRNA in PBMC were significantly increased compared with controls. A possible interpretation of this finding is that this elevation is compensating the decrease in the AE2 expression.

CONCLUSIONS AND QUESTIONS FOR THE FUTURE

From all these data, we may conclude that AE2 is the AE protein specifically expressed in the liver. Its presence at the luminal membrane in both hepatocytes and cholangiocytes strongly suggests that AE2 is the carrier involved in choride/bicarbonate exchange in the hepatobiliary tract, and therefore in the transport of bicarbonate to the bile as well as in the formation of ductular bile. In line with this is the finding that transcriptional expression of AE2 appears to be more intense in cholangiocytes than in hepatocytes. Liver expression of the AE2 gene has been found to be decreased in PBC patients compared with patients with normal liver and individuals with cirrhosis and cholestasis other than PBC. This impaired AE gene expression has been detected at both the mRNA and the protein level. Additional evidence for a widespread alteration of AE2 expression in PBC was obtained in PBC lymphocytes having lower AE2 mRNA levels than controls, and in salivary glands from PBC patients with sicca syndrome showing a decreased AE2 immunoreactivity. Based on these data, we can speculate that abnormal AE2 gene expression may participate in the pathogenesis of PBC playing a role in: (a) decreased production of ductular bile and cholestasis; (b) pluriglandular exocrine failure; (c) disturbed regulation of intracellular pH which may cause altered cell function and antigenicity in BEC, and immunoreactivity changes in lymphocytes; and (d) alteration of acid–base transport in a variety of tissues which may contribute to other systemic disturbances, such as osteodystrophy by affecting osteoclast function.

A number of questions remain for the future regarding the role of AE2 in PBC: is abnormal AE2 expression a primary event in PBC?; is it a phenomenon secondary to other endocrine, immunologic, or metabolic alterations occurring in this disease?; does it reflect a more complex and basic defect in systems controlling gene expression? Much research is needed to disclose the pathogenesis of a disease which still remains an enigma.

References

1. Leung PS, Van-de-Water J, Coppel RL, Nakanuma Y, Munoz S, Gershwin ME. Molecular aspects and the pathological basis of primary biliary cirrhosis. J Autoimmun 1996;9:119–28.
2. Joplin R, Gershwin ME. Ductular expression of autoantigens in primary biliary cirrhosis. Semin Liver Dis 1997;17:97–103.
3. Goddard GJR, Warnes TW. Primary biliary cirrhosis: how should we evaluate new treatments? Lancet 1994;343:1305–6.
4. Alper SL. The band 3-related AE anion exchanger gene family. Cell Physiol Biochem 1994;4:265–81.
5. Prieto J, Qian C, García N, Díez J, Medina JF. Abnormal expression of anion exchanger genes in primary biliary cirrhosis. Gastroenterology 1993;105:572–8.
6. García C, Montuenga LM, Medina JF, Prieto J. In situ detection of AE2 anion-exchanger mRNA in the human liver. Cell Tissue Res 1998;291:481–8.
7. Martínez-Ansó E, Castillo JE, Díez J, Medina JF, Prieto J. Immunohistochemical detection of chloride/bicarbonate anion exchangers in human liver. Hepatology 1994;19:1400–6.
8. Strazzabosco M. New insights into cholangiocyte physiology. J Hepatol 1997;27:945–52.
9. Medina JF, Martínez-Ansó E, Vázquez JJ, Prieto J. Decreased anion exchanger 2 immunoreactivity in the liver of patients with primary biliary cirrhosis. Hepatology 1997;25:12–17.
10. Vázquez JJ, Vázquez M, Idoate MA, et al. Anion exchanger immunoreactivity in human salivary glands in health and Sjögren's syndrome. Am J Pathol 1995;146:1422–32.

6
Molecular considerations of primary biliary cirrhosis

M. E. GERSHWIN, C. T. MIGLIACCIO, J. VAN DE WATER AND R. L. COPPEL

INTRODUCTION

Primary biliary cirrhosis is a destructive autoimmune disease of the intra-hepatic bile ducts characterized by inflammation of the portal triads, fibrosis and the presence of antimitochondrial antibodies[1,2]. The typical patient with PBC is 40–60 years of age, female, with a clinical presentation of lethargy, pruritus that is debilitating and persistent, or mild jaundice. PBC is virtually the only autoimmune disease never reported in a pediatric population, and is uncommon before age 30, after which the incidence gradually rises with age. Increasingly, however, patients are being detected in the presymptomatic stage as a result of multiphasic laboratory screening tests because of eleva-tions in serum alkaline phosphatase. The pathological changes in PBC are best thought of as an autoimmune cholangiolitis and the common scheme of histological grading of severity recognizes four stages[3].

Antimitochondrial antibodies (AMA), found in 90–95% of patients with PBC, are a major criterion for diagnosis of the disease. Approximately 5–10% of patients with PBC do not have serum AMA; yet the clinical and histological findings of AMA-positive and AMA-negative patients do not differ significantly. It has been suggested in the past that antibodies to mitochondrial antigens in sera of patients with PBC arise simply as a response to hepatocyte and bile ductular injury. Recent data extensively contradict this idea and support the concept that PBC is a 'model' auto-immune disease[4–6]. First, the highly directed and high-titer response to PDC-E2 are unique to PBC and are typical of what is found in other organ-specific autoimmune diseases[7]. Second, the absence of such antibodies in patients or animals with chronic biliary obstruction and/or infection with *Escherichia coli* implies that AMAs are not merely a response to recurrent cholangitis[8,9]. Third, the constellation of a predominance of T cells found in lesions, the presence of immune complexes, the primary involvement of biliary ductular cells and the results of an *in-vitro* study of autoantibody production suggests that a target antigen is involved[10-16]. Fourth, the similarity of the pathology of PBC to chronic graft-versus-host disease suggests that the injury is immunologically mediated[17]. Fifth, the reported recurrence of PBC in some patients after liver transplantation accords with the concept that PBC is indeed an organ-specific autoimmune disease[18-22].

AMA AND THEIR AUTOANTIGENS

Extensive effort has been devoted to the characterization of the antimitochondrial autoantibody response by patients with PBC. Several distinct characteristics have been documented. Firstly, the major reactivity appears to be with PDC-E2. Serum autoantibodies from 90-95% of patients with PBC react with PDC-E2 by immunoblotting or ELISA[23-26], whereas the frequency of reactivity against E2 subunits of OGDC and BCOADC is lower, around 50-70%[2,27]. A single patient may have reactivity against several mitochondrial autoantigens, but with the exception of PDC-E2 and protein X (E3BP), each autoantigen is recognized by a distinct population of autoantibodies[28]. Secondly, epitope mapping data suggest a paucity of B cell epitopes on the autoantigens[29-31]. In the case of PDC-E2, there is a major epitope encompassing residues 128-221, the inner lipoyl domain. Autoantibodies also react to residues 1-90, the outer lipoyl domain, but at a one hundred-fold lower dilution. Given the sequence similarity between the two regions, this observation has been interpreted as indicative of cross-reactivity between the two lipoyl domains[29]. AMA have very potent inhibitory effects on the *in-vitro* catalytic activity of the enzyme with which they react[30-35]. It is noteworthy that antibodies are almost totally non-inhibitory with purified bacterial PDC, despite the reactivity of sera with both enzymes by immunoblotting. These findings indicate that there is a fine antigenic difference in the lipoyl domains of the mammalian and bacterial enzymes. Furthermore, the extent of the antimitochondrial response is variable but can be extremely high with specific titers to PDC-E2 using dilutions of sera in the hundreds of thousands or millions.

Antimitochondrial antibodies are the hallmark of PBC. Although it is not clear that AMA are involved in the pathogenesis of the disease, the study of these autoantibodies has enabled a great deal of information to be learned about the specificity of this response. Prior to the identification of the major mitochondrial antigens of PBC as components of the 2-oxo acid dehydrogenase enzyme family, mitochondrial antigens were believed to be extremely diverse and were divided into nine subtypes termed M1-M9. This classification was based upon data derived from the relatively non-specific biochemical and immunological techniques that were available[36]. The M2 antigen is now known to correspond to the 2-oxo acid dehydrogenase enzymes. The pivotal development in the study of PBC was the cloning and identification of the autoantigen targets for antimitochondrial antibodies[23,25,37,38]. However, it was not until the last decade that the targets of those antibodies were characterized. It was discovered that AMA from patients with PBC reacted to this complex located on the inner mitochondrial membrane. The first antigen isolated from this complex was PDC-E2. The breakthrough

Table 1 Summary of the mitochondrial autoantigens of PBC

Antigen	Molecular weight (kDa)	Complex	Cloned	T epitope identified	B epitope identified
PDC-E2	74	PDC	+	+	+
BCOADC-E2	52	BCOADC	+	−	+
OGDC-E2	48	OGDC	+	−	+
Protein X (E3BP)	56	PDC	−	−	−
PDC-E1α	41	PDC	+	−	+
PDC-E1β	36	PDC	+	−	−

Table 2 Characteristic features of the antimitochondrial response in PBC

	Autoantibody			
	PDC-E2	BCOADC-E2	OGDC-E2	E1α
Localization of the major B cell epitope	Inner lipoyl domain	Inner lipoyl domain	Inner lipoyl domain	TPP binding site
Amino acid residues	128–221	No distinct binding subregion	67–147	NA
Predominant Ig class and isotype	IgG3 and IgM	NA	IgG2 and IgM	NA
Inhibitory effect on the in-vitro enzyme catalytic activity	+	+	+	+
Percentage of reactivity according to ethnic background				
Japanese	15/23 (65%)*	16/23 (70%)	11/23 (48%)	11/23 (47%)
American Caucasian	37/39 (95%)*	17/23 (73%)	12/39 (31%)	9/23 (39%)
Murine monoclonal antibodies				
V_{H} gene usage	Diverse array of V_{H} gene segments	NA	NA	NA
Human combinatorial antibodies				
V_{H} gene usage	Clonally related heavy chains displaying a high number of somatic mutations	NA	NA	NA

TPP: thiamine pyrophosphate.
* Statistically significant difference ($p = 0.0037$, Fisher's exact test).

came in 1987 when a cDNA for the 74-kDa mitochondrial autoantigen was cloned and sequenced[37], leading to identification of the major autoantigen as the E2 component of the mitochondrial pyruvate dehydrogenase complex (PDC)[32,39]. Subsequently, a group of antigens associated with PDC and related enzymes were identified as components of a functionally related enzyme family, the 2-oxo acid dehydrogenase complexes (2-OADC) of which PDC is the most prominent antigenic component[23,24,26,32–35,37,39].

The elucidation of the three major complexes involved in the autoantibody response of PBC took over a decade, beginning with PDC-E2 being sequenced in the mid-1980s[37] and culminating with the epitope mapping and reactivity to the OGDC complex subunits in the mid-1990s[40]. The first work was done almost exclusively on the PDC-E2 subunit. The fact that AMA in almost all PBC sera reacted with this protein, as described above, explains the reason for this focus. In early mapping studies, it was found that the antibodies recognized, and inhibited, the functional site of the enzyme[23]. Similar data were produced by studies of the BCOADC enzymes when they were mapped with patient sera[33]. Consistent with this is the observation that many autoimmune sera inhibit the function of their target antigens[23,41]. Several studies have suggested that autoantigens relevant to PBC may be present on the surface of hepatocytes or biliary epithelium. PBC sera react with the surface of teased-out hepatocytes and intact hepatoma cells; such reactivity is abolished by prior absorption of sera with mitochondria[42]. Interestingly, there is a skewed distribution of class and isotype of autoantibodies with a predominance of IgG_3 and IgM[43,44].

The complex of mitochondrial proteins focused upon in the study of PBC has been characterized mostly by reaction to sera from patients with PBC. The major mitochondrial autoantigen, PDC-E2, which has an apparent molecular weight of 74 kDa, is the E2 component, dihydrolipoamide acetyltransferase, of the pyruvate dehydrogenase complex[25,37]. The 56-kDa mitochondrial autoantigen is protein X (E3BP) of pyruvate dehydrogenase. It possesses crossreactive epitopes with the 74-kDa antigen. The 52-kDa mitochondrial autoantigen is the equivalent E2, dihydrolipoamide acetyltransferase of BCOADC[45]. The 48-kDa antigen is the equivalent E2 component of α-ketoglutarate (OGDC-E2). The fifth (common) and sixth (uncommon) mitochondrial autoantigens are PDC-E1α and PDC-E1β; these proteins, unlike the antigens above, do not contain lipoic acid[34]. These results and data on cloning of the other autoantigens are shown in Tables 1 and 2.

The immunodominant epitope of PDC-E2 was localized to the lipoic-acid-binding site of the rat PDC-E2. Human PDC-E2, in contrast to rat PDC-E2, has two lipoic-acid-binding sites. By using a full-length human cDNA for PDC-E2, and by preparation of multiple overlapping recombinant fragments, we have determined that three autoreactive determinants are present on human PDC-E2: two crossreactive lipoyl domains, and an area surrounding the E1/E3 binding region. By probing small restriction fragments of the inner lipoyl domain, it is believed that the autoepitope includes a conformational component. The major epitope is within the region surrounding the inner lipoyl domain[25,29]. The advent of cDNAs for mitochondrial autoantigens has allowed not only for more precise studies of their role in PBC but also for the development of rapid and sensitive immunoassays.

The epitope recognized by AMA specific to BCOADC-E2 in PBC has been mapped by taking advantage of a full-length BCOADC-E2 cDNA and a series of expression clones spanning the entire molecule. Reactivity to 12 expression clones was studied by immunoblotting, ELISA, and selective absorption of patient sera by expressed protein fragments. Autoantibodies to BCOADC-E2 map within peptides spanning amino-acid residues 1–227 of the mature protein; our data demonstrate that the epitope is dependent on conformation and includes the lipoic-acid-binding region[46]. Similarly, data on selective absorption of anti-BCOADC-E2 activity by 19 expressing clones is in production. Moreover, the absence of lipoic acid on the recombinant polypeptides used in this study indicates that antibody binding to BCOADC-E2 is not dependent on the presence of lipoic acid[46].

The E2 subunit of the 2-oxoglutarate dehydrogenase complex, dihydrolipoamide succinyltransferase (OGDC-E2), is another of the mitochondrial autoantigens being studied for PBC. Eighty out of 268 (29.9%) PBC patient sera tested reacted with an OGDC-E2 recombinant fusion protein, but none of the sera obtained from autoimmune hepatitis, primary sclerosing cholangitis (PSC), systemic lupus erythematosus (SLE) or normals. A series of overlapping recombinant peptides spanning the entire OGDC-E2 molecule were constructed and probed with sera from patients with PBC. Results indicate that a minimum of 81 amino acid residues (67–147) which correspond to the OGDC-E2 inner lipoyl domain were required for reactivity. In addition, the flanking regions of the lipoyl domain augmented this response. These results suggest that the OGDC-E2 B cell epitope is also conformational. Furthermore, absorption of PBC sera with the recombinant OGDC-E2 peptide specifically removed reactivity to OGDC-E2 but not PDC-E2 and BCOADC-E2, demonstrating that there appears to be no crossreactivity between this OGDC-E2 epitope, PDC-E2 or BCOADC-E2 molecules (unpublished data).

Each of the 2-oxo acid dehydrogenase complexes are located on the mammalian inner mitochondrial membrane and include PDC, the 2-oxoglutarate dehydrogenase complex (OGDC), and the branched-chain 2-oxo acid dehydrogenase (BCOADC)[45]. Each complex consists of three subunits, E1, E2, and E3; all are nuclear-encoded proteins that are separately imported into mitochondria for assembly into high-molecular-weight multimers on the inner membrane[47]. In each case, the predominant antibody reactivity to the enzyme complex is against the E2 component, which is a lipoamide acetyltransferase for the PDC and BCOADC, and a succinyl transferase for the OGDC[23,33,34,46]. In the case of the pyruvate dehydrogenase complex, there are two additional complex components that are autoantigens, protein X (E3BP) and E1[35,38]. It is believed that protein X (E3BP) reacts by virtue of the presence of a crossreactive epitope between PDC-E2 and protein X (E3BP); almost all anti-PDC-E2 antibody reagents recognize protein X (E3BP) and no patient serum has been identified with anti-protein X (E3BP) reactivity without concomitant anti-PDC-E2 reactivity[38].

Simultaneous examination of liver sections with an anti-isotype reagent for human IgA revealed high IgA staining in the luminal region of biliary epithelial cells in patients with PBC. Apical staining by mAbs to mito-chondrial antigens has been observed and will be discussed below. IgG and IgA antibodies to PDC-E2 were detected in the bile of patients with PBC but not normal controls[48]. These data have been independently confirmed by Joplin et al.[49,50]; they reported that cultured biliary epithelial cells from PBC patients have luminal surface membrane-bound PDC-E2. Further, the British group has used transmission electron microscopy to demonstrate that the staining is on the surface of BEC[51]. They used two antibodies which recognized PDC-E2, affinity-purified rabbit anti-PDC-E2 and affinity-purified human (PBC) anti-PDC-E2, for their localization studies. Both antibodies also bound to the inner membrane of mitochondria in BEC isolated from patients with PBC and controls. However, binding to the external aspect of the plasma membrane was observed only in BEC from patients with PBC.

OTHER AUTOANTIBODIES AND THEIR ANTIGENS

Nuclear antigens

There are two different staining patterns, by immunofluorescence, with regard to antinuclear autoantibodies in patients with PBC. One is the 'multiple nuclear dot' pattern and the other is referred to as the 'nuclear rim' pattern. The difference between these two patterns was discovered to be recognition of intranuclear proteins versus that of the nuclear envelope. The intranuclear proteins recognized by patient sera have been found to be Sp100 and the PML protein[52]. Sp100 is an acidic phosphorylated nuclear protein with a molecular weight of 53 kDa, while PML was identified as a nuclear matrix-associated protein containing structural features consistent with transcriptional regulatory proteins. While these two have been found to colocalize, experiments have not revealed any direct interaction between them. For the antibodies that recognize antigens of the nuclear envelope, there are two types: a 'smooth' staining pattern versus a 'punctate' staining pattern[53]. The 'smooth' pattern corresponds to antibodies that recognize the lamin B receptor (LBR). While antibodies to LBR have been isolated from only a few patients with PBC, they have not been reported in any other disease. The 'punctate' staining of the nuclear envelope corresponds to antibodies that recognize nuclear pore complexes[53,54]. There are two antigens that have been isolated: gp210 and p62. Up to 20% of patients with PBC have been found to have antibodies to gp210, while a larger number have been reported with anti-p62 antibodies. These autoantibodies are not as prevalent in patients with PBC as the AMA. They are found in about 25% of the AMA-positive patients with PBC, but in close to 100% of AMA-negative subjects. Not all who are AMA-negative have antibodies for every nuclear protein but they do tend to have at least one.

Other antigens

In addition to the above mentioned autoantibody responses seen in patients with PBC, antibodies to platelets have likewise been detected. In one study, about 40% of the patients produced detectable levels of platelet antibodies[55]. It is not clear whether the thrombocytopenia seen in patients with PBC is immune mediated, and whether or not it is isolated to this one auto-immune disease.

LUMINAL STAINING

Sera from patients with PBC react with enzymes of the 2-oxo dehydrogenase pathway, particularly PDC-E2. These enzymes are present in all nucleated cells, yet autoimmune damage is confined to biliary epithelial cells. Using a panel of monoclonal antibodies and a human combinatorial antibody specific for PDC-E2, sections of liver from patients with PBC, PSC and hepatocarcinoma were initially examined by indirect immunofluorescence and confocal microscopy. The monoclonal antibodies gave typical mito-chondrial immunofluorescence on biliary epithelium and on hepatocytes from patients with either PBC, PSC or hepatocarcinoma. However, 1 of 8 mouse monoclonal antibodies (C355.1) reacted with great intensity and specificity with the luminal region of biliary epithelial cells from patients with PBC. Using pixel intensity analysis, quantification of these differences was possible. We believe that these data may be interpreted as indicating that either a PDC-E2 fragment or a molecule crossreactive with PDC-E2 is present in high concentrations in the luminal region of biliary epithelial cells in PBC[48,56].

The polyclonal nature of AMA and the limited success of generating human mAb have made analysis of fine specificity and antibody hetero-geneity difficult. To address the relative importance of the region(s) within the inner lipoyl domain to antibody binding, detailed profiles of 12 PDC-E2-specific combinatorial antibodies (Fabs SP1 through SP12) have been performed. The Fabs react specifically to PDC-E2 with high affinity ($K_a = 10^{-7}–10^{-10}$ mol/L^{-1}) and recognize a conformational epitope within the inner lipoyl domain. Furthermore, the antibodies demonstrate heterogeneity with substantial differences in relative recognition of different recombinant PDC-E2 fragments and differential recognition patterns against mutant constructs of the human PDC-E2 inner lipoyl domain (amino acid residues 91–227). In addition, five of the Fab clones (SP1, 3, 4, 8 and 12) demonstrate different staining patterns on biliary epithelial cells of patients with PBC but not with control liver disease. Some of the Fabs specifically stained the apical region of biliary epithelium, a pattern distinct from typical mito-chondrial staining and again a pattern specific for PBC. Immunoglobulin gene sequencing suggests that the IgG anti-PDC-E2 repertoire of PBC patients is the result of the clonal expansion of a restricted set of B-cells[57,58].

It has been demonstrated that a molecule crossreactive with PDC-E2 is expressed at high levels in the luminal region of biliary epithelial cells in PBC. This abnormal staining is not found in other tissues in patients with

PBC, with the exception of some PBC salivary gland epithelium. The salivary glands of control patients, including Sjögren's syndrome, are normal[59]. Examination of liver biopsies was performed using confocal microscopy and pixel intensity histogram analysis following staining with C355.1, SP4, or control mAb, for abnormal luminal/apical staining of BEC. Interestingly, 7/9 AMA-negative patients had abnormal staining of their BEC, in a manner similar to AMA-positive patients. We will not repeat the data as they have already been discussed as well as published[48]. C355.1 has also been used to stain sections of liver from both a patient with PBC and a control patient (PSC). The result was an intense staining in the apical region in PBC only. A similar profile is seen with the human combinatorial SP4 in PBC but not PSC. The only staining seen with C355.1 or SP4 in the control liver is in the cytoplasmic region, consistent with mitochondria. Additional controls, including use of other antibodies and other tissues, have been published[48,56,57,59]; data from the UK demonstrating that the PDC-E2 staining is on the cell surface have been discussed above[49,50,60] and will be further evaluated in our longitudinal study.

Our laboratory has extended these data by studying the binding of murine monoclonal and human combinatorial phage autoantibodies to BEC of patients with PBC and controls[48,57]. These antibodies, specific for PDC-E2, all produce, as expected, positive immunofluorescence of mitochondria when used to stain HEp-2 cells[61]. However, in our first study, 1 of 8 mouse monoclonal antibodies (C355.1) and a human combinatorial antibody also reacted with great intensity and specificity with the luminal region of biliary epithelial cells from patients with PBC. We postulated that the selective reactivity of some anti-PDC-E2 reagents may be interpreted as indicating that a molecule crossreactive with PDC-E2 is expressed at high levels in the luminal region of biliary epithelial cells in PBC. Subsequently, we demonstrated that expression of this molecule precedes the presence of both MHC class II and BB1/B7 on biliary epithelial cells[62].

RECOMBINANT ANTIGENS

Like many other processes studied, recombinants have opened many doors of possibilities for researchers. Once the mitochondrial antigens recognized in PBC were isolated and sequenced, recombinant proteins were utilized for furthering the study of the disease. Recombinant antigens have been used in various capacities in the study of PBC. One of the original uses was in the screening of patient sera for AMA. First, individual antigens (PDC-E2, etc.) were utilized, and later a hybrid protein consisting of the lipoyl domains of each E2 subunit from the three complexes (PDC, BCOADC, and OGDC) was created. The use of recombinant fusion proteins and designer 'hybrid' molecules provides a reliable and rapid assay for quantitation of AMA and is highly diagnostic of PBC. Immunoassays have facilitated the examination for Ig subclass restriction shown to exist for antibodies to PDC-E2, BCOADC-E2, and PDC-E1α[24,35,43,46,62]. These recombinant proteins were also used to produce mAbs. These monoclonals were then characterized (antigen recognition, tissue staining) in the hope of elucidating the pathogenesis of this disease. The results have been the discovery of mAbs specific for the other subunits (OGDC and BCOADC) that produce apical staining of BEC in tissue sections from patients with PBC and not PSC.

OTHER DISEASES

Autoantibody reactivity to the mitochondrial autoantigens in PBC exhibit several features that are similar to many autoimmune diseases. The autoantigens are intracellular enzymes and these enzymes are part of multiprotein complexes such as the splicing machinery in SLE or Sjögren's syndrome or the mitochondrial complexes in PBC[63–66]. The antibodies can be present in very high titer and show reactivity against the target autoantigen in several species, i.e. the autoepitopes are conserved in evolution and are likely to be functionally important parts of the molecule[67–69]. This is less commonly observed using animal sera raised against autoantigens; this observation has been used to suggest that there is something special about the event of tolerance breakdown that focuses responsiveness to regions of the molecule that are normally immunologically silent. A major difference between PBC and other autoantibody responses is that, for other well-studied diseases, the autoantibodies detect several epitopes within the target antigen, i.e. U1RNP[70] in mixed connective tissue disease and La in Sjögren's syndrome[71]. The implication from these studies is that the autoantibody response is 'antigen driven', i.e. it has been induced by the target antigen itself. In contrast, there appears to be only a single, although somewhat long, autoepitope in PDC-E2 and this raises the possibility that the initial response was raised against another protein, a 'molecular mimic', and the autoantigen is recognized by virtue of a crossreactive response.

FUTURE

The pathogenesis of PBC is still unknown, as it is for the other organ-specific autoimmune diseases. Infection by microorganisms containing constituent molecules that induce an immune response that crossreacts with self has been suggested as a causative event. In support of this 'molecular mimicry' is the observation that the structure of the family of E2 transacylases is conserved among species and crossreactivity of AMA from PBC patients to microbial mitochondrial proteins has been reported[72,73]. For such a hypothesis to be tenable it needs to explain the origin of the polyspecific responses to several different proteins. Were all of these present as separate molecular mimics in the original infecting organism, or did these responses arise subsequently with some general loss of tolerance to a number of proteins? It has been suggested that a PDC-E2-like molecule was the original mimic, as this is the most commonly recognized autoepitope and because of the unexpected apical staining of some anti-PDC-E2 antibodies on biliary epithelium from patients with PBC[48]. The responses to other antigens were suggested to have arisen after the original breaking of tolerance perhaps by a mechanism of determinant spreading or by some form of crossreactivity[5]. Attempts have been made to examine this hypothesis further by searching for crossreactivity between mitochondrial autoantigens and by examining the repertoire of immunoreactive species in PBC tissue. Although it has been shown that a subset of AMA react with more than one mitochondrial antigen[74], detailed studies about such AMA crossreactivity using well-defined molecular reagents have been lacking.

As with any area of research, the more that is discovered, the more questions are raised. Now that the antigen targets of PBC AMA have been discovered, do we understand their role(s)? Are they causes or results of the disease? Are AMA, the hallmark of PBC, recognizing self proteins or is it some crossreactive epitope or molecular mimic? Based on the conserved nature of the mitochondrial proteins, there is a possibility of this type of molecular mimicry in PBC. This could be coupled with the spreading of determinants recognized by the immune system in the initial infection to further encompass a reaction to self proteins. But how does this explain two things?: localization of destruction to the BEC, and recognition of proteins that should not be encountered by the immune system. And what of the other autoantibodies discovered in patients with PBC? While found in some, but not all patients, what is their role, if any?

Some future directions in the study of this disease will be the elucidation of the epitope being recognized on the apical surface of BEC and its origin. If this is not a protein-specific response but, rather a crossreactive conformational epitope, then the mapping of it might shed some light on the origins of the AMA response in PBC and, hopefully, the destruction of the bile ducts. Unfortunately, we are not at the level of protein research where a conformational epitope can be easily sent through a bank of sequences to find a match. This works well for linear epitopes but not 3-dimensional ones. The discovery of additional reactivities located in the target tissue of the disease and crossreacting with the targets of AMA opens several new avenues for investigation into the etiology of this disease.

References

1. Kaplan MM, Knox TA. Treatment of primary biliary cirrhosis with low-dose weekly methotrexate. Gastroenterology 1991;101:1332–8.
2. Gershwin ME, Mackay IR. Primary biliary cirrhosis: paradigm or paradox for autoimmunity. Gastroenterology 1991;100:822–33.
3. Dickson ER, Fleming CR, Ludwig J. Primary biliary cirrhosis. Prog Liv Dis 1979;6:487–502.
4. James SP, Hoofnagle JH, Strober W, et al. NIH conference: Primary biliary cirrhosis: a model autoimmune disease. Ann Intern Med 1983;99:500–12.
5. Coppel RL, Gershwin ME. Primary biliary cirrhosis: The molecule and the mimic. Immunol Rev 1995;144:17–49.
6. Leung PS, Van de Water J, Coppel RL, et al. Molecular characterization of the mitochondrial autoantigens in primary biliary cirrhosis. Immunol Res 1991;10:518–27.
7. Leung PS, Krams S, Munoz S, et al. Characterization and epitope mapping of human monoclonal antibodies to PDC-E2, the immunodominant autoantigen of primary biliary cirrhosis. J Autoimmun 1992;5:703–18.
8. Krams SM, Surh CD, Coppel RL, et al. Immunization of experimental animals with dihydrolipoamide acetyltransferase, as a purified recombinant polypeptide, generates mitochondrial antibodies but not primary biliary cirrhosis. Hepatology 1989;9:411–16.
9. Lever E, Balasubramanian K, Condon S, et al. Primary biliary cirrhosis associated with ulcerative colitis. Am J Gastroenterol 1993;88:945–7.

10. Van de Water J, Ansari A, Prindiville T, et al. Heterogeneity of autoreactive T cell clones specific for the E2 component of the pyruvate dehydrogenase complex in primary biliary cirrhosis. J Exp Med 1995;181:723-33.
11. Karlsson-Parra A, Nyberg A, Totterman TH, et al. Primary biliary cirrhosis – phenotypic characterization of immunocompetent cells in peripheral blood and liver tissue. Uppsala J Med Sci 1984;89:254-65.
12. Bjorkland A, Festin R, Mendel-Hartvig I, et al. Blood and liver-infiltrating lymphocytes in primary biliary cirrhosis: increase in activated T and natural killer cells and recruitment of primed memory T cells. Hepatology 1991;13:1106-11.
13. Bjorkland A, Totterman TH. Is primary biliary cirrhosis an autoimmune disease? Scand J Gastroenterol Suppl 1994;204:32-9.
14. Van de Water J, Ansari AA, Surh CD, et al. Evidence for the targeting by 2-oxo-dehydro-genase enzymes in the T cell response of primary biliary cirrhosis. J Immunol 1991;146: 89-94.
15. Lohr H, Fleischer B, Gerken G, et al. Autoreactive liver-infiltrating T cells in primary biliary cirrhosis recognize inner mitochondrial epitopes and the pyruvate dehydrogenase complex. J Hepatol 1993;18:322-7.
16. Leon MP, Spickett G, Jones DE, et al. CD4+ T cell subsets defined by isoforms of CD45 in primary biliary cirrhosis. Clin Exp Immunol 1995;99:233-9.
17. Vierling JM. Immune disorders of the liver and bile duct. Gastroenterol Clin N Am 1992;21:427-49.
18. Weaver GA, Franck WA, Streck WF. Recurrence of primary biliary cirrhosis after liver transplantation. N Engl J Med 1982;306:1235-6.
19. Wong PY, Portmann B, O'Grady JG, et al. Recurrence of primary biliary cirrhosis after liver transplantation following FK506-based immunosuppression. J Hepatol 1993;17:284-7.
20. Neuberger J, Portmann B, Macdougall BR, et al. Recurrence of primary biliary cirrhosis after liver transplantation. N Engl J Med 1982;306:1-4.
21. Dietze O, Vogel W, Margreiter R, et al. Early recurrence of primary biliary cirrhosis after liver transplantation. Gastroenterology 1990;98:1106-7.
22. Hart J, Busuttil RW, Lewin KJ. Disease recurrence following liver transplantation. Am J Surg Pathol 1990;1:79-91.
23. Van de Water J, Gershwin ME, Leung P, et al. The autoepitope of the 74-kD mitochondrial autoantigen of primary biliary cirrhosis corresponds to the functional site of dihydrolipoa-mide acetyltransferase. J Exp Med 1988;167:1791-9.
24. Van de Water J, Cooper A, Surh CD, et al. Detection of autoantibodies to recombinant mitochondrial proteins in patients with primary biliary cirrhosis. N Engl J Med 1989;320:1377-80.
25. Coppel RL, McNeilage LJ, Surh CD, et al. Primary structure of the human M2 mito-chondrial autoantigen of primary biliary cirrhosis: dihydrolipoamide acetyltransferase. Proc Natl Acad Sci USA 1988;85:7317-21.
26. Fussey SP, Guest JR, James OF, et al. Identification and analysis of the major M2 autoanti-gens in primary biliary cirrhosis. Proc Natl Acad Sci USA 1988;85:8654-8.
27. Mackay IR, Gershwin ME. Primary biliary cirrhosis: current knowledge, perspectives, and future directions. Semin Liv Dis 1989;9:149-57.
28. Mackay IR, Gershwin ME. Primary biliary cirrhosis: considerations on pathogenesis based on identification of the M2 autoantigens. Semin Immunopathol 1990;12:101-19.
29. Surh CD, Coppel R, Gershwin ME. Structural requirement for autoreactivity on human pyruvate dehydrogenase-E2, the major autoantigen of primary biliary cirrhosis. Implication for a conformational autoepitope. J Immunol 1990;144:3367-74.
30. Sundin U. Antibody binding and inhibition of pyruvate dehydrogenase (PDH) in sera from patients with primary biliary cirrhosis. Clin Exp Immunol 1990;81:238-43.
31. Uibo R, Mackay IR, Rowley M, et al. Inhibition of enzyme function by human autoantibod-ies to an autoantigen pyruvate dehydrogenase E2: different epitope for spontaneous human and induced rabbit autoantibodies. Clin Exp Immunol 1990;80:19-24.
32. Van de Water J, Fregeau D, Davis P, et al. Autoantibodies of primary biliary cirrhosis recognize dihydrolipoamide acetyltransferase and inhibit enzyme function. J Immunol 1988;141:2321-4.
33. Fregeau DR, Davis PA, Danner DJ, et al. Antimitochondrial antibodies of primary biliary cirrhosis recognize dihydrolipoamide acyltransferase and inhibit enzyme function of the branched chain alpha-ketoacid dehydrogenase complex. J Immunol 1989;142:3815-20.

34. Fregeau DR, Prindiville T, Coppel RL, et al. Inhibition of alpha-ketoglutarate dehydrogenase activity by a distinct population of autoantibodies recognizing dihydrolipoamide succinyltransferase in primary biliary cirrhosis. Hepatology 1990;11:975–81.
35. Fregeau DR, Roche TE, Davis PA, et al. Primary biliary cirrhosis. Inhibition of pyruvate dehydrogenase complex activity by autoantibodies specific for E1 alpha, a non-lipoic acid containing mitochondrial enzyme. J Immunol 1990;144:1671–6.
36. Berg PA, Klein R. Autoantibodies in primary biliary cirrhosis. Springer Semin Immunopathol 1990;12:85–99.
37. Gershwin ME, Mackay IR, Sturgess A, et al. Identification and specificity of a cDNA encoding the 70 kd mitochondrial antigen recognized in primary biliary cirrhosis. J Immunol 1987;138:3525–31.
38. Surh CD, Roche TE, Danner DJ, et al. Antimitochondrial autoantibodies in primary biliary cirrhosis recognize crossreactive epitope(s) on protein X and dihydrolipoamide acetyltransferase of pyruvate dehydrogenase complex. Hepatology 1989;10:127–33.
39. Yeaman SJ, Fussey SP, Danner DJ, et al. Primary biliary cirrhosis: identification of two major M2 mitochondrial autoantigens. Lancet 1988;1:1067–70.
40. Moteki S, Leung P, Dickson E, et al. Epitope mapping and reactivity of autoantibodies to the E2 component of 2-oxoglutarate dehydrogenase complex in primary biliary cirrhosis using recombinant 2-oxoglutarate dehydrogenase complex. Hepatology 1996;23(3):436–44.
41. Imai H, Fritzler MJ, Neri R, et al. Immunocytochemical characterization of human NOR-90 (upstream binding factor) and associated antigens reactive with autoimmune sera. Two MR forms of NOR-90/hUBF autoantigens. Mol Biol Rep 1994;19:115–24.
42. Ghadiminejad I, Baum H. Evidence for the cell-surface localization of antigens crossreacting with the 'mitochondrial antibodies' of primary biliary cirrhosis. Hepatology 1987;7:743–9.
43. Surh CD, Cooper AE, Coppel RL, et al. The predominance of IgG3 and IgM isotype antimitochondrial autoantibodies against recombinant fused mitochondrial polypeptide in patients with primary biliary cirrhosis. Hepatology 1988;8:290–5.
44. Outschoorn I, Rowley MJ, Cook AD, et al. Subclasses of immunoglobulins and autoantibodies in autoimmune diseases. Clin Immunol Immunopathol 1993;66:59–66.
45. Surh CD, Danner DJ, Ahmed A, et al. Reactivity of primary biliary cirrhosis sera with a human fetal liver cDNA clone of branched-chain alpha-keto acid dehydrogenase dihydrolipoamide acyltransferase, the 52 kDa mitochondrial autoantigen. Hepatology 1989;9:63–8.
46. Leung PSC, Chuang DT, Wynn RM, et al. Autoantibodies to BCOADC-E2 in patients with primary biliary cirrhosis recognize a conformational epitope. Hepatology 1995;22:505–13.
47. Yeaman SJ. The mammalian 2-oxoacid dehydrogenases: a complex family. Trends Biochem Sci 1986;11:293–7.
48. Van de Water J, Turchany J, Leung PS, et al. Molecular mimicry in primary biliary cirrhosis. Evidence for biliary epithelial expression of a molecule crossreactive with pyruvate dehydrogenase complex-E2. J Clin Invest 1993;91:2653–64.
49. Joplin R, Lindsay JG, Hubscher SG, et al. Distribution of dihydrolipoamide acetyltransferase (E2) in the liver and portal lymph nodes of patients with primary biliary cirrhosis: an immunohistochemical study. Hepatology 1991;14:442–7.
50. Joplin R, Lindsay JG, Johnson GD, et al. Membrane dihydrolipoamide acetyltransferase (E2) on human biliary epithelial cells in PBC. Lancet 1992;339:93–4.
51. Joplin R, Wallace LL, Johnson GD, et al. Subcellular localization of pyruvate dehydrogenase dihydrolipoamide acetyltransferase in human intrahepatic biliary epithelial cells. J Pathol 1995;175.
52. Szostecki C, Guldner HH, Will H. Autoantibodies against 'nuclear dots' in primary biliary cirrhosis. Semin Liv Dis 1997;17:71–8.
53. Courvalin JC, Worman HJ. Nuclear envelope protein autoantibodies in primary biliary cirrhosis. Semin Liv Dis 1997;17:79–90.
54. Miyachi K, Shibata M, Onozuka Y, et al. Primary biliary cirrhosis sera recognize not only gp210 but also proteins of the p62 complex bearing N-acetylglucosamine residues from rat liver nuclear envelope. Mol Biol Rep 1996;23:227–34.
55. Feistauer SM, Penner E, Mayr WR, et al. Target platelet antigens of autoantibodies in patients with primary biliary cirrhosis. Hepatology 1997;25:1343–5.
56. Cha S, Leung PS, Coppel RL, et al. Heterogeneity of combinatorial human autoantibodies against PDC-E2 and biliary epithelial cells in patients with primary biliary cirrhosis. Hepatology 1994;20:574–83.

57. Pascual V, Cha S, Gershwin ME, *et al.* Nucleotide sequence analysis of natural and combinatorial anti-PDC-E2 antibodies in patients with primary biliary cirrhosis. Recapitulating immune selection with molecular biology. J Immunol 1994;152:2577–85.
58. Tsuneyama K, Van de Water J, Nakanuma Y, *et al.* Human combinatorial autoantibodies and mouse monoclonal antibodies to PDC-E2 produce abnormal apical staining of salivary glands in patients with coexistent primary biliary cirrhosis and Sjögren's syndrome. Hepatology 1994;20:893–8.
59. Joplin RE, Johnson GD, Matthews JB, *et al.* Distribution of pyruvate dehydrogenase dihydrolipoamide acetyltransferase (PDC-E2) and another mitochondrial marker in salivary gland and biliary epithelium from patients with primary biliary cirrhosis. Hepatology 1994;19:1375–80.
60. Cha S, Leung PS, Gershwin ME, *et al.* Combinatorial autoantibodies to dihydrolipoamide acetyltransferase, the major autoantigen of primary biliary cirrhosis. Proc Natl Acad Sci USA 1993;90:2527–31.
61. Tsuneyama K, Van de Water J, Leung PSC, *et al.* Abnormal expression of the E2 component of the pyruvate dehydrogenase complex on the luminal surface of biliary epithelium occurs before major histocompatibility complex class II and BB1/B7 expression. Hepatology 1995;21:1031–7.
62. Surh CD, Ahmed-Ansari A, Gershwin ME. Comparative epitope mapping of murine monoclonal and human autoantibodies to human PDH-E2, the major mitochondrial autoantigen of primary biliary cirrhosis. J Immunol 1990;144:2647–52.
63. McNeilage LJ, Umapathysivam K, Macmillan E, *et al.* Definition of a discontinuous immunodominant epitope at the NH2 terminus of the La/SS-B ribonucleoprotein autoantigen. J Clin Invest 1992;89:1652–6.
64. Ben-Chetrit E. The molecular basis of the SSA/Ro antigens and the clinical significance of their autoantibodies. Br J Rheumatol 1993;32:396–402.
65. Frank MB, McCubbin VR, Heldermon C. Expression and DNA binding of the human 52 kDa Ro/SSA autoantigen. Biochem J 1995;305:359–62.
66. Huff JP, Roos G, Peebles CL, *et al.* Insights into native epitopes of proliferating cell nuclear antigen using recombinant DNA protein products. J Exp Med 1990;172:419–29.
67. Troster H, Metzger TE, Semsei I, *et al.* One gene, two transcripts: isolation of an alternative transcript encoding for the autoantigen La/SS-B from a cDNA library of a patient with primary Sjögren's syndrome. J Exp Med 1994;180:2059–67.
68. Talal N, Garry RF, Schur PH, *et al.* A conserved idiotype and antibodies to retroviral proteins in systemic lupus erythematosus. J Clin Invest 1990;85:1866–71.
69. O'Brien RM, Cram DS, Coppel RL, *et al.* T-cell epitopes on the 70-kDa protein of the (U1)RNP complex in autoimmune rheumatologic disorders. J Autoimmun 1990;3:747–57.
70. McNeilage LJ, Macmillan EM, Whittingham SF. Mapping of epitopes on the La(SS-B) autoantigen of primary Sjögren's syndrome: identification of a crossreactive epitope. J Immunol 1990;145:3829–35.
71. Bassendine MF, Fussey SPM, Mutimer DJ, *et al.* Identification and characterization of four M2 mitochondrial autoantigens in primary biliary cirrhosis. Semin Liv Dis 1989;9:124–31.
72. Morreale M, Tsirigotis M, Hughes MD, *et al.* Significant bacteriuria has prognostic significance in primary biliary cirrhosis. J Hepatol 1989;9:149–58.
73. Flannery GR, Burroughs AK, Butler P, *et al.* Antimitochondrial antibodies in primary biliary cirrhosis recognize both specific peptides and shared epitopes of the M2 family of antigens. Hepatology 1989;10:370–4.
74. Fusconi M, Baum H, Caselli A, *et al.* Demonstration of peptide-specific and cross-reactive epitopes in proteins reacting with antimitochondrial antibodies of primary biliary cirrhosis. J Hepatol 1992;15:162–9.

7
Animal models of primary biliary cirrhosis

C. D. HOWELL, J. LI AND W. CHEN

INTRODUCTION

PBC fulfills four of the five criteria for an autoimmune disease (Table 1), but the etiology and immunopathogenesis of PBC are not well defined. A better understanding of the mechanisms responsible for bile duct destruction and hepatic fibrosis during chronic non-suppurative destructive cholangitis may lead to more effective medical therapies for this disease. However, several factors hamper the capacity to address these questions in patients. The onset of PBC is obscured by an initial preclinical/asymptomatic stage that lasts up to 20 years. Consequently, advanced stage III (fibrosis) or stage IV (cirrhosis) liver pathology is present in 50% of subjects at the time of diagnosis. In addition, the functions of T cells freshly isolated from established lesions cannot be assessed, since percutaneous liver biopsy specimens do not yield adequate numbers of cells for *in-vitro* studies. Also, whether the T cells cloned from the livers of patients with established PBC are representative of the primary T cells that initiate destruction of intrahepatic bile ducts and hepatic fibrosis *in vivo* is unclear. Moreover, MHC-matched or autologous intrahepatic bile duct cells are not available to directly examine how T cells mediate destruction of intrahepatic bile duct cells. These obstacles have led to increasing interest in animal models of PBC.

Table 1   PBC: autoimmune?

- Circulating antibody or cell-mediated immunity to an autoantigen
- Definition of the specific autoantigen
- Disease transferred to experimental animal by autoantibody or self-reactive cells (?)
- Disease induction in experimental animal by immunization with the autoantigen (No)
- Generation of autoantibody or self-reactive cells by immunizing experimental animal with autoantigen

Table 2 Animal models of NSDC

Spontaneous
  Rabbits, Faenza Italy*
  Senescent female C57BL/6 mouse
Human-SCID mouse*
Immunization with syngeneic or allogeneic bile duct cells (rat and mouse)
Immunization with pyruvate dehydrogenase
Inoculation with mycoplasma-like organisms, CD-1 mouse
IL2 mouse gene knockout
Mdr2 (P-glycoprotein) mouse gene knockout
Graft-versus-host disease

---

* Anti-mitochondrial antibodies

An ideal animal model of PBC would have the following attributes:

(a) The onset and course of NSDC would be highly reproducible;
(b) The immunophenotypes of infiltrating liver inflammatory cells (CD4+, $\alpha\beta$ T cells $\geq$ CD8+ $\alpha\beta$ T cells) and intrahepatic bile duct epithelial cells (aberrant MHC class II and ICAM 1 expression) and hepatic lymphokine profiles (bias toward pro-inflammatory Th1) in fully developed liver lesions would be similar to PBC;
(c) The liver lesions would progress to fibrosis and cirrhosis;
(d) Animals would develop serum antimitochondrial antibodies with a high frequency.

Non-suppurative destructive cholangitis (NSDC) has been reported in many laboratory animal species (Table 2). However, no model appears to reproducibly progress to cirrhosis, and the frequency of serum antimitochondrial (and anti-bile duct) antibodies has been highly variable. Furthermore, except for the mouse GVHD models described below, most models have not been validated by independent investigators and the pathogenesis of NSDC has not been examined in detail.

SPONTANEOUS MODELS OF NSDC

In 1982, Tison *et al.* reported PBC-like lesions in a domestic rabbit model identified in Faenza, Italy[1]. Cirrhosis developed in some animals. Approximately 50% of affected rabbits exhibited serum antimitochondrial antibodies. However, this rabbit model is no longer available. Hayashi *et al.* reported NSDC lesions in 60% of female and male C57BL/6 mice over 2 years of age[2]. The hepatic lesions in this model are accompanied by inflammatory lesions in salivary and thyroid glands, lungs, pancreas, and kidneys. Serum anti-bile duct cell antibodies are detected in 14% of mice. However, the liver lesions in this model have not been further characterized.

HUMAN SCID MOUSE MODELS

In an attempt to develop a mouse model of PBC, two groups of investigators transferred human peripheral blood cells isolated from PBC patients or human controls into immunodeficient SCID mice[3,4]. In both studies, mice reconstituted with PBC-lymphocytes developed human M2 antimito-chondrial antibodies. Krams et al. observed NSDC lesions in 64% of mice injected with PBC peripheral blood cells[3]. By comparison, Abedi et al. detected no abnormalities in liver histology in their human PBC–SCID mouse studies. The explanation for these contradictory results is unknown. However, Krams found NSDC in 20% of SCID mice reconstituted with normal human control cells[3], raising the possibility that the lesions were due to a graft-versus-host reaction to xenogeneic mouse antigens.

IMMUNIZATION WITH INTRAHEPATIC BILE DUCT CELLS

Ueno et al. induced NSDC and anticholangiocyte antibodies in Wistar/HD rats by immunization with syngeneic rat intrahepatic bile duct cells in Freund's complete adjuvant (CFA)[5]. The liver lesions persisted for 1–6 weeks after onset, and were reproduced by booster immunizations. Spleen cells isolated from this model transferred NSDC to syngeneic rats and lysed syngeneic cholangiocytes (but not hepatocytes) in vitro. This observation suggests that bile duct cell death in this model is mediated by cytotoxic T cells that recognize bile-duct-specific antigens. Alternatively, bile duct cells may have a greater capacity to present endogenous antigens to sensitized T cells than hepatocytes. PBC-like liver lesions developed in 64% of neonatal thymectomy A/J (H-2K) mice following immunization with xenogeneic (pig) intrahepatic bile duct cells[6]. The liver inflammatory infiltrate included T and B cells, and intrahepatic bile ducts expressed aberrant MHC class II molecules. Serum M2-AMA (anti-PDH E2) were detected in 42% of mice.

INOCULATION WITH PYRUVATE DEHYDROGENASE (PDH), PURIFIED PDH-E2, OR INFECTIOUS MATERIALS

A cardinal principle of an autoimmune disease is the capacity to generate the lesion(s) in an experimental animal model by immunization with the identified autoantigen. Immunization of BALB/c mice with the PDH-E2 antigen leads to the production of antibodies to PDH-E2, but immunized animals do not exhibit liver pathology[7]. Others have induced NSDC lesions in female C57BL/6 mice by inoculation with bacterial LPS, purified PDH, and CFA[8]. Inflammatory changes were also observed in the livers of control mice injected with CFA and PDH/CFA or LPS/CFA. Therefore, the extent to which the lesions in this model represent specific reactivity to PDH is unknown. Johnson detected NSDC with granulomatous inflammation and portal fibrosis in mice inoculated subcutaneously with vitreous tissue from patients with chronic intraocular inflammation due to mycoplasma-like organisms[9]. However, the liver lesions were infrequent, occurring in only 11 of 100 mice.

GENE KNOCKOUT MICE

NSDC has been reported in mice made to be deficient in interleukin (IL-2) and the mdr2 P-glycoprotein by gene targeting[10,11]. IL-2-deficient (IL-$2^{-/-}$)

129/Ola × C57Bl/6 mice develop intestinal lesions reminiscent of chronic ulcerative colitis, anti-colon antibodies, and anemia between 4 and 9 weeks of age[12]. In contrast, IL-2$^{-/-}$ BALB/c mice do not exhibit colonic inflammation, but show generalized autoimmunity with hemolytic anemia, pancreatitis, pulmonary vasculitis, myocarditis, NSDC, and death by 5 weeks of age. Spleen, lymph node, and bone marrow T cells isolated from IL-2$^{-/-}$ mice show an activated phenotype that appears to be important to disease expression. The functions and antigen specificity of T cells isolated from the liver have not been examined. Investigation of this model may identify the process through which a genetically determined immune dysfunction (IL-2 deficiency) leads to the maturation of autoreactive T and B cells and intrahepatic bile duct damage.

The mdr2 (homolog of human MDR3) gene encodes a protein that is critical to the transport of phospholipids into bile across the hepatocyte canalicular membrane. In mdr2 (P-glycoprotein) gene knockout mice, NSDC occurs shortly after birth and progresses to maximum levels between 3 and 6 months[11]. Biliary phospholipid concentrations are negligible and biliary glutathione and cholesterol concentrations are markedly diminished. Yet, bile flow is increased to 2–3 times the normal rate. These animals exhibit elevated serum bilirubins and ultrastructural changes in the hepatic canaliculus consistent with cholestasis. Subsequently, mdr$^{-/-}$ animals develop multifocal primary hepatocellular carcinoma that becomes metastastic around 15 months of age. This model suggests that a primary defect in biliary phospholipid secretion and bile formation may lead to NSDC and hepatic carcinogenesis, though the specific mechanisms have not been established.

GRAFT-VERSUS-HOST DISEASE (GVHD) MODELS

PBC-like lesions have been described in many laboratory animal models of GVHD. However, the large number of well-defined inbred congeneic, and recombinant strains have made the mouse models particularly popular for studying the T cell subpopulations, costimulatory and adhesion molecules, and lymphokines that mediate GVHD. In all models, GVHD is dependent on the presence of mature (competent) $\alpha\beta$ T cells in the graft that recognize foreign transplantation antigens (major histocompatibility (MHC) class I and II, MHC class II, and/or non-MHC or minor histocompatibility antigens) expressed in a host that is incapable of rejecting the graft. Depending on the donor and host strains and the nature of the alloantigen disparity, GVHD may be either acute (associated with strong donor antihost CTL activity, immunosuppression to third party alloantigens, and high mortality) or chronic (low mortality, weak antihost CTL activity, autoimmune-like features). In general, GVHD directed at allogeneic MHC class I antigens tends to be acute and dependent on donor CD8+ (MHC class I-restricted; cytotoxic/suppressor) cells, while GVHD directed at host MHC class II antigens is dependent on donor CD4+ (MHC class II-restricted; helper) cells. GVHD across a full MHC (class I and II) tends to involve both subsets and is frequently dependent on donor CD4+ cells. Either donor CD4+ or

CD8 donor T cells may independently mediate NSDC across multiple minor histocompatibility (non-MHC) antigens depending on the donor and host[13-15]. Moreover, NSDC (and cutaneous GVHD) has been observed in rats and mice that have been irradiated and reconstituted with syngeneic (self) bone marrow. In the syngeneic GVHD models, radiation injury to the host thymus appears to interfere with negative selection (deletion) of self-reactive T cells, leading to autoimmune lesions in the skin and liver. However, the targeted autoantigens have not been determined.

We have focused on the B10.D2 into irradiated BALB/c mouse GVHD model[16-22]. Analogous to GVHD in human recipients of HLA-matched bone marrow transplantation, the donor and host strains in this mouse model are MHC-identical ($H-2^d$) and differ at multiple minor histocompatibility (miH) or non-MHC alloantigens and Mls 3, a viral superantigen encoded by mouse mammary tumor virus-6 and recognized by donor $V\beta3+$ cells. The course of NSDC is highly reproducible in this model, progressing from mild portal inflammation 3 days after transplantation of donor spleen cells to marked inflammation and NSDC between day 14 and 42. Subsequently, the liver lesions resolve spontaneously. This model also exhibits cutaneous lesions, and marked elevations in serum IgE concentrations typical of chronic GVHD in humans[23,24]. The intrahepatic bile ducts and portal vein endothelial cells in this model express aberrant MHC class II and ICAM 1 molecules beginning between day 3 and 7 after transplantation. Lymphocytes isolated from the liver also produce a variety of T lymphokines with a bias toward interferon γ, a pro-inflammatory Th1 cytokine (Chen et al., submitted). Donor CD4+ cells are dominant in the liver of the host during the 7–10 days after transplantation, but donor CD8+ cells predominate between days 14 and 42[18,19]. However, NSDC in this GVHD model is dependent on donor CD4 cells (Figure 1)[17]. Indeed, naive donor CD4 cells are capable of mediating hepatic GVHD in the absence of liver CD8+ cells. Donor CD8+ cells are not essential and also are unable to mediate hepatic lesions in the absence of donor CD4+ cells. All told, our results indicate that NSDC in this GVHD model is induced by donor CD4 (MHC class II-restricted) cells that recognize miHC antigens presented by BALB/c host APC. Activated donor CD4+ cells subsequently mediate NSDC through two pathways. A fundamental pathway is independent of donor CD8 T cells. An auxiliary pathway appears to involve CD4-dependent, donor CD8 (MHC class I-restricted) cells. The functions of liver-infiltrating CD4+ and CD8+ effector T cells and the mechanisms responsible for damage to intrahepatic bile duct cells in this model are the subject of ongoing studies.

To further explore the T cells and antigens that mediate the liver lesions in this model, we examined the β chain variable region ($V\beta$) repertoire used by donor CD4 and CD8 cells isolated from the mature liver lesions on day 14 through 40 after transplantation[19]. Each mouse with GVHD had at least one expanded $V\beta$ population in the liver but there was considerable variability between individual mice. Yet, CD4+ isolated from the liver during GVHD preferentially used T cell receptors $V\beta2$ and $V\beta3$ (Figure 2A). $V\beta2+$ and $V\beta3+$ CD4+ cells were expanded in the livers of 65% and 88% of mice with GVHD, respectively. The $V\beta$ repertoire used by liver CD8+ cells

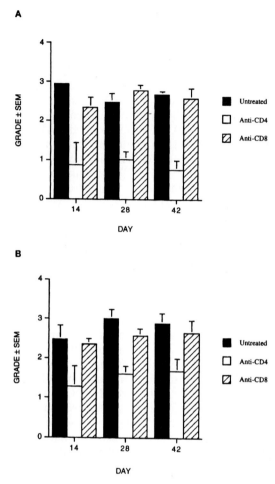

Figure 1 Effect of anti-CD4 and anti-CD8 treatments on liver histology and serum IgE levels during murine GVHD. GHVD mice were treated intraperitoneally with either anti-CD4 ($n=28$) or anti-CD8 ($n=27$) on days 0 and 7 or days 0, 7, 14, and 21. Control GVHD mice ($n=29$) received no treatment. Mice were killed on days 14, 28, and 42 after the last dose of antibody. Liver specimens were stained with hematoxylin and eosin. Coded slides were analyzed for the portal tract inflammation (A) and bile duct lesion (B) scores using criteria outlined in ref. 17. Results from ≥3 separate experiments were pooled and expressed as the mean grade ±SEM. $p<0.005$(A) and $p<0.01$ (B), anti-CD4 vs. untreated and anti-CD8 treated mice on each day.
Reproduced from Transplantation 1996; 62: 1621–1628 by permission of the publishers.

was less biased, but expansion of Vβ8+ cells was most impressive (Figure 2B). No mice showed expansion of self (auto)-reactive Vβ5+ and 11+ cells in the liver during NSDC. Vβ2+ CD4 cells were increased preferentially in the liver compared with the spleen (data not shown). Thus, we hypothesized that expanded Vβ2+ cells are a large oligoclonal popula-

A

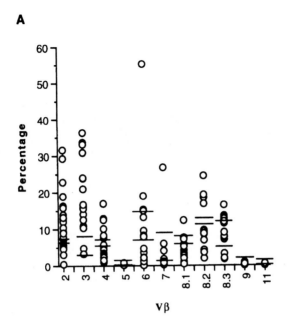

B

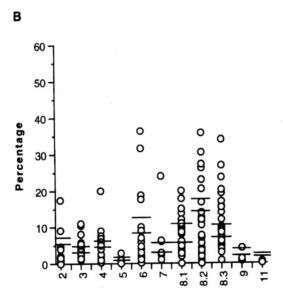

Figure 2 Summary of TCR Vβ repertoires in GVHD mice. Analysis of Vβ repertoire was performed as described in Figure 2. Numbers of mice studied for Vβ2, 3, 4, 5, 6, 7, 8.1, 8.2, 8.3, 9, and 11 populations were (A), Liver CD4 cells: 23, 17, 19, 7, 24, 9, 14, 14, 14, 7, and 6, respectively; (B), Liver CD8 cells:15, 20, 14, 5, 19, 8, 28, 28, 28, 3, and 3, respectively. The horizontal bars show the mean percentage ± 2 SD for normal B10,D2 CD4 (A) or CD8 (B) cells. Reproduced from The Journal of Immunology 1995; 155: 2350–8 by permission of the publishers.

tion that might recognize a liver-specific alloantigen. If so, Vβ2 TCR would be homologous in the third complementarity-determining region (CDR3), the TCR β chain residues that bind to conventional peptide antigens bound to MHC class II molecules. In contrast, we speculated that expansion of Vβ3+ cells in the liver and spleen is driven by recognition of Mls 3, a viral superantigen expressed in BALB/c (host) mice. Thus, we predicted that Vβ3+ cells are polyclonal with respect to conventional peptide antigen specificity and contain highly diverse CDR3 regions. Using RT-PCR, we found a limited TCR Vβ repertoire (Vβs 1, 2, 3, 4, 6, and 8) in the liver on day 3 during the initiation of NSDC (Chen et al., submitted). Furthermore, to analyze the clonal nature of liver Vβ2+ and Vβ3+ cells, we determined the nucleotide and amino acid sequences of the CDR3 regions in liver Vβ2 and Vβ3 libraries prepared from individual mice with GVHD on days 3 and 14. We found that both liver Vβ2+ and Vβ3+ T cells undergo clonal expansion in the liver during the first 2 weeks NSDC, consistent with specific recognition of a 1–3 dominant host miHC antigen(s) in the liver of each mouse. Leibnitz et al. have also reported that a large number of CD4+ T cells (hybridomas) propagated from the liver of the B6 into (bm1 × bm12)F1 (MHC class I and II disparity) are specific for host alloantigens[25].

Studies of antigen-specific T cell clones in vitro have shown costimulation through CD28:B7-1 (CD80)/B7-2 (CD86) is critical for T cell activation. Stimulation of T cell clones with antigen:MHC in the absence of this costimulatory signal leads to T cell anergy. However, Dubey et al. have shown that either CD80/CD86 or ICAM-1 (CD54) can provide sufficient costimulation to activate naive, resting T cells[26]. Recent studies indicate that the nature of the costimulatory molecules expressed by APC can determine the patterns of lymphokine produced by T cells[27–30]. Death rates in mice with acute GVHD have been decreased considerably by in-vivo treatments that block costimulatory T cell signals through LFA-1a (CD11a):ICAM-1 (CD54), CD28/cytotoxic T lymphocyte-associated molecule (CTLA)4:B7-1 (CD80)/B7-2 (CD86), and VLA-4 (CD29d):vascular cell adhesion molecule (VCAM)-1, and CD40:CD40 ligand[31–37]. However, the hepatic lesions of GVHD persisted in one mouse acute GVHD model following treatment with CTLA4-Ig fusion protein (blockade of CD80/CD86) despite protection from GVHD mortality[37]. These results suggest that other costimulatory receptor:ligand systems may be able to substitute for CD80/CD86 during initiation of NSDC in vivo. Howell et al. (manuscript submitted) have reported that anti-ICAM 1 suppress NSDC in the B10.D2 into BALB/c mouse GVHD model. Likewise, Kimura et al. have reported that antibodies directed to epitopes in the α chain of LFA 1 (CD11a/CD18) suppresses PBC-like lesions and serum antimitochondrial antibody production in vivo in the B6 into (B6 × bm12) GVHD model directed to host MHC class II antigens[38].

The clinical manifestations of GVHD in some mouse models appear to be correlated with the profile of lymphokines produced by donor T cells activated in the spleen[39–41]. For example, spleen cells isolated from the B6→BDF1 acute GVHD model preferentially produce pro-inflammatory

Th1 (IL-2, IFNγ, lymphotoxin) lymphokines during the first 2 weeks after transplantation. Acute GVHD in this model results in potent anti-host CTL activity, increased serum IgG2a levels, and high mortality rates. By comparison, spleen cells isolated from the lupus-like, DBA/2 → BDF1 chronic GVHD model preferentially produce IL-4 and IL-10 (Th2). This chronic GVHD model develops serum IgG1 and IgG2b autoantibodies and immune complex glomerulonephritis, associated with weak antihost CTL activity and low death rates. Williamson et al. have shown that IL-12, a cytokine that promotes Th1 cell differentiation and IFNγ production, is critical to the acute GVHD[40]. And Via et al. have reported that treatment of DBA/2 → BDF1 mice with IL-12 also leads to acute GVHD[39]. Treatment of some acute murine GVHD models with pharmacological doses of purified lymphokines or neutralizing antibodies to cytokines has ameliorated or prevented death due to acute GVHD, demonstrating an important role for lymphokines in the induction of GVHD[42-45]. And treatment of the BALB/c → CBF1 chronic GVHD model with anti-IL-4 prevented hepatic lesions as well as elevation in serum IgE levels[46]. These studies suggest that IL-4 (a Th2 lymphokine) is critical to hepatic and humoral features of chronic GVHD in this particular model, challenging the notion that pro-inflammatory lymphokines are required for tissue inflammation. The requirement for particular Th1 and Th2 lymphokines during NSDC in other animal models has not been determined.

SUMMARY

There is no natural animal model of PBC. Several animal models of non-suppurative destructive cholangitis have been reported though none of them mimic all the full spectrum of hepatic histopathology, serological abnormalities, and extrahepatic lesions associated with PBC. Yet, overall, these models indicate that a variety of mechanisms (immune dysfunction due to IL-2 deficiency, mdr2 P-glycoprotein deficiency) and antigens (infections, autologous, allogeneic, and xenogeneic) may be involved in the pathogenesis of NSDC. There is a critical need for more extensive investigations of the antigens, hepatic effector cells, costimulatory molecules, and lymphokines/soluble mediators that mediate bile duct destruction in the various models of NSDC. Systematic studies of these models may provide new insights into the etiology and pathogenesis of chronic NSDC in patients with PBC.

References

1. Tison V, Callea F, Morisi C, et al. Spontaneous 'primary biliary cirrhosis' in rabbits. Liver 1982;2(2):152–61.
2. Hayashi Y, Utsuyama M, Kurashima C, Hirokawa K. Spontaneous development of organ-specific autoimmune lesions in aged C57BL/6 mice. Clin Exp Immunol 1989;78:120–6.
3. Krams SM, Dorshkind K, Gershwin ME. Generation of biliary lesions after transfer of human lymphocytes into severe combined immunodeficient (SCID) mice. J Exp Med 1989;170(6):1919–30.
4. Abedi MR, Hammarstrom L, Broome U, et al. Reduction in serum levels of antimito-chondrial (M2) antibodies following immunoglobulin therapy in severe combined immuno-

deficient (SCID) mice reconstituted with lymphocytes from patients with primary biliary cirrhosis (PBC). Clin Exp Immunol 1996;105(2):266–73.

5. Ueno Y, Phillips JO, Ludwig J, et al. Development and characterization of a rodent model of immune-mediated cholangitis. Proc Natl Acad Sci USA 1996;93(1):216–20.

6. Kobayashi H, Yamamoto K, Yoshioka T, et al. Nonsuppurative cholangitis is induced in neonatally thymectomized mice: A possible animal model of primary biliary cirrhosis. Hepatology 1994;19(6):1424–30.

7. Krams SM, Surh CD, Coppel RL, et al. Immunization of experimental animals with dihydrolipoamide acetyltransferase, as a purified recombinant polypeptide, generates mitochondrial antibodies but not primary biliary cirrhosis. Hepatology 1989;9(3):411–16.

8. Ide T, Sata M, Suzuki H, et al. An experimental animal model of primary biliary cirrhosis induced by lipopolysaccharide and pyruvate dehydrogenase. Kurume Med J 1996; 43(3):185–8.

9. Johnson L, Wirostko E, Wirostko W. Primary biliary cirrhosis in the mouse: induction by human mycoplasma-like organisms. Int J Exp Pathol 1990;71(5):701–12.

10. Sadlack B, Lohler J, Schorle H, et al. Generalized autoimmune disease in interleukin-2-deficient mice is triggered by an uncontrolled activation and proliferation of CD4+ T cells. Eur J Immunol 1995;25(11):3053–9.

11. Mauad TH, van Nieuwkerk CM, Dingemans KP, et al. Mice with homozygous disruption of the mdr2 P-glycoprotein gene. A novel animal model for studies of nonsuppurative inflammatory cholangitis and hepatocarcinogenesis. Am J Pathol 1994;145(5):1237–45.

12. Sadlack B, Merz H, Schorle H, et al. Ulcerative colitis-like disease in mice with a disrupted interleukin-2 gene [see comments]. Cell 1993;75(2):253–61.

13. Williams FH, Thiele DL. The role of major histocompatibility complex and non-major histocompatibility complex encoded antigens in generation of bile duct lesions during hepatic graft-vs.-host responses mediated by helper or cytotoxic T cells. Hepatology 1994;19(4):980–8.

14. Murphy GF, Whitaker D, Sprent J, Korngold R. Characterization of target injury of murine acute graft-versus-host disease directed to multiple minor histocompatibility antigens elicited by either CD4+ or CD8+ effector cells. Am J Pathol 1991;138(4):983–90.

15. Okunewick JP, Kociban DL, Buffo MJ. Comparative effects of various T cell subtypes on GVHD in a murine model for MHC-matched unrelated donor transplant. Bone Marrow Transplant 1990;5(3):145–52.

16. Onishi S, Saibara T, Nakata S, et al. Cytotoxic activity of spleen-derived T lymphocytes against autologous biliary epithelial cells in autopsy patients with primary biliary cirrhosis. Liver 1993;13(4):188–92.

17. Li J, Helm K, Howell CD. Contributions of donor CD4 and CD8 cells to murine hepatic graft-versus-host disease. Transplantation 1996;62(11):1621–8.

18. Howell CD, De Victor D, Li J, et al. Liver T cell subsets and adhesion molecules in murine graft-versus-host disease. Bone Marrow Transplant 1995;16(1):139–45.

19. Howell CD, Li J, Roper E, Kotzin BL. Biased liver T cell receptor V beta repertoire in a murine graft-versus-host disease model. J Immunol 1995;155(5):2350–8.

20. Howell CD, Yoder TY, Vierling JM. Suppressor function of liver mononuclear cells isolated during murine chronic graft-vs-host disease. II. Role of prostaglandins and interferon-gamma. Cell Immunol 1992;140(1):54–66.

21. Howell CD, Yoder TD, Vierling JM. Suppressor function of hepatic mononuclear inflammatory cells during murine chronic graft-vs-host disease. I. Macrophage-enriched cells mediate suppression in the liver. Cell Immunol 1991;132(1):256–68.

22. Howell CD, Yoder T, Claman HN, Vierling JM. Hepatic homing of mononuclear inflammatory cells isolated during murine chronic graft-vs-host disease. J Immunol 1989; 143(2):476–83.

23. Claman HN, Jaffee BD, Huff JC, Clark RA. Chronic graft-versus-host disease as a model for scleroderma. II. Mast cell depletion with deposition of immunoglobulins in the skin and fibrosis. Cell Immunol 1985;94(1):73–84.

24. Claman HN, Spiegelberg HL. Immunoglobulin dysregulation in murine graft-vs-host disease: a hyper-IgE syndrome. Clin Immunol Immunopathol 1990;56(1):46–53.

25. Leibnitz RR, Lipsky PE, Thiele DL. Reactivity of hybridomas derived from T cells activated in vivo during graft-versus-host disease. J Immunol 1994;153(11):4959–68.

26. Dubey C, Croft M, Swain SL. Costimulatory requirements of naive CD4+ T cells. ICAM-1 or B7-1 can costimulate naive CD4 T cell activation but both are required for optimum response. J Immunol 1995;155(1):45–57.
27. Croft M, Swain SL. Recently activated naive CD4 T cells can help resting B cells, and can produce sufficient autocrine IL-4 to drive differentiation to secretion of T helper 2-type cytokines. J Immunol 1995;154(9):4269–82.
28. McArthur JG, Raulet DH. CD28-induced costimulation of T helper type 2 cells mediated by induction of responsiveness to interleukin 4. J Exp Med 1993;178(5):1645–53.
29. Petro TM, Chen SS, Panther RB. Effect of CD80 and CD86 on T cell cytokine production. Immunol Invest 1995;24(6):965–76.
30. Shanafelt MC, Soderberg C, Allsup A, et al. Costimulatory signals can selectively modulate cytokine production by subsets of CD4+ T cells. J Immunol 1995;154(4):1684–90.
31. Blazar BR, Taylor PA, Panoskaltsis-Mortari A, et al. Blockade of CD40 ligand–CD40 interaction impairs CD4+ T cell-mediated alloreactivity by inhibiting mature donor T cell expansion and function after bone marrow transplantation. J Immunol 1997;158(1):29–39.
32. Blazar BR, Sharpe AH, Taylor PA, et al. Infusion of anti-B7.1 (CD80) and anti-B7.2 (CD86) monoclonal antibodies inhibits murine graft-versus-host disease lethality in part via direct effects on CD4+ and CD8+ T cells. J Immunol 1996;157(8):3250–9.
33. Korngold R. Lethal graft-versus-host disease in mice directed to multiple minor histocompatibility antigens: features of CD8+ and CD4+ T cell responses. Bone Marrow Transplant 1992;9(5):355–64.
34. Wallace PM, Johnson JS, MacMaster JF, et al. CTLA4Ig treatment ameliorates the lethality of murine graft-versus-host disease across major histocompatibility complex barriers. Transplantation 1994;58(5):602–10.
35. Schlegel PG, Vaysburd M, Chen Y, et al. Inhibition of T cell costimulation by VCAM-1 prevents murine graft-versus-host disease across minor histocompatibility barriers. J Immunol 1995;155(8):3856–65.
36. Blazar BR, Taylor PA, Panoskaltsis-Mortari A, et al. Coblockade of the LFA1:ICAM and CD28/CTLA4:B7 pathways is a highly effective means of preventing acute lethal graft-versus-host disease induced by fully major histocompatibility complex-disparate donor grafts. Blood 1995;85(9):2607–18.
37. Blazar BR, Taylor PA, Linsley PS, Vallera DA. In vivo blockade of CD28/CTLA4: B7/BB1 interaction with CTLA4-Ig reduces lethal murine graft-versus-host disease across the major histocompatibility complex barrier in mice. Blood 1994;83(12):3815–25.
38. Kimura T, Suzuki K, Inada S, et al. Monoclonal antibody against lymphocyte function-associated antigen 1 inhibits the formation of primary biliary cirrhosis-like lesions induced by murine graft-versus-host reaction. Hepatology 1996;24(4):888–94.
39. Via CS, Rus V, Gately MK, Finkelman FD. IL-12 stimulates the development of acute graft-versus-host disease in mice that normally would develop chronic, autoimmune graft-versus-host disease. J Immunol 1994;153(9):4040–7.
40. Williamson E, Garside P, Bradley JA, Mowat AM. IL-12 is a central mediator of acute graft-versus-host disease in mice. J Immunol 1996;157(2):689–99.
41. Rus V, Svetic A, Nguyen P, et al. Kinetics of Th1 and Th2 cytokine production during the early course of acute and chronic murine graft-versus-host disease. Regulatory role of donor CD8+ T cells. J Immunol 1995;155(5):2396–406.
42. Krenger W, Snyder K, Smith S, Ferrara JL. Effects of exogenous interleukin-10 in a murine model of graft-versus-host disease to minor histocompatibility antigens. Transplantation 1994;58(11):1251–7.
43. Krenger W, Snyder KM, Byon JC, et al. Polarized type 2 alloreactive CD4+ and CD8+ donor T cells fail to induce experimental acute graft-versus-host disease. J Immunol 1995;155(2):585–93.
44. Sykes M, Szot GL, Nguyen PL, Pearson DA. Interleukin-12 inhibits murine graft-versus-host disease. Blood 1995;86(6):2429–38.
45. Fowler DH, Kurasawa K, Smith R, et al. Donor CD4-enriched cells of Th2 cytokine phenotype regulate graft-versus-host disease without impairing allogeneic engraftment in sublethally irradiated mice. Blood 1994;84(10):3540–9.
46. Ushiyama C, Hirano T, Miyajima H, et al. Anti-IL-4 antibody prevents graft-versus-host disease in mice after bone marrow transplantation. The IgE allotype is an important marker of graft-versus-host disease. J Immunol 1995;154(6):2687–96.

8
Fibrogenesis in PBC

D. SCHUPPAN AND E. G. HAHN

PBC IS A PROGRESSIVE FIBROGENIC DISORDER

Classical PBC is characterized by ongoing destruction of portal and interlobular bile ducts which often leads to cirrhosis. Patients with symptomatic disease usually progress in a predictable manner, allowing timely referral for liver transplantation. Although a subgroup of asymptomatic patients who show only moderate but typical laboratory and histological abnormalities may not progress significantly over one or two decades[1,2], many patients will develop cirrhosis within a few years. Thus, progression from histological stage I (portal inflammation; $n = 15$) and stage II (portal and periportal inflammation; $n = 56$) to stage IV (cirrhosis) after 4 years reached 30% and 50%, respectively, in a single center[3]. Since development of cirrhosis is the major determinant affecting survival in patients with PBC and since the etiology of the disease is little understood, therapeutic strategies that are based on a better knowledge of the mechanisms of fibrogenesis in PBC would be helpful.

MECHANISMS OF FIBROGENESIS

Liver fibrogenesis, i.e. the excess synthesis and deposition of extracellular matrix (ECM), can be initiated by several triggers. Such triggers are hepatotoxins, hepatotropic viruses, immune reactions to the liver, metabolic diseases, and biliary stasis. In acute liver diseases, such as viral hepatitis A, fibrogenesis is balanced by fibrolysis, i.e. the removal of excess ECM. However, with a repeated insult of sufficient severity, as in many chronic liver diseases, fibrogenesis outweighs fibrolysis, finally resulting in morphologically apparent fibrosis or cirrhosis. Usually, damage to the hepatocyte or the bile duct epithelium leads to mononuclear cell activation, release of fibrogenic factors and activation of mesenchymal cells. In this scenario, the activated Kupffer cell and the macrophage are thought to be the primary sources of potentially fibrogenic cytokines and growth factors[4-9], whereas the hepatic stellate cell (the novel denomination for the perisinusoidal lipocyte or Ito cell) and the portal fibroblast have been identified as the cell types that are responsible for excess ECM deposition in the liver[5,6,8–11]. Both cell types have their correlates in other mesenchymal–epithelial organs, like the skin, the kidney, the lung and the intestine, that are susceptible to fibrosis[12–14]. Upon activation by fibrogenic growth factors and disruption of their three-dimensional ECM environment, these usually quiescent cells undergo a transformation into a contractile myofibroblastic phenotype with high proliferative potential and the capacity to produce an excess of ECM molecules. This reflects a protective program, aimed at rapid closure of a potentially lethal wound[14,15], which is self-limited if the offending agent is present for a short period of time but leads to fibrosis and cirrhosis when continuously activated.

THE ROLE OF BILE DUCT EPITHELIAL CELLS IN FIBROGENESIS

Classical histology as well as more recent immunological, cell and molecular biological studies suggest that bile duct epithelial cells (BDEC) play a key role in the fibrogenesis of PBC as well as of secondary biliary fibrosis:

(a) Bile duct lesions, either as the mononuclear cell infiltration of early stages or as the proliferating bile ductules of later stages, are a hallmark of the disease;

(b) Active collagen expression occurs in apparently freshly recruited myofibroblastic cells around *de-novo* formed bile ductules as can be shown by markers of mesenchymal activation[16] and by *in-situ* hybridization[17,18];

(c) Proliferating BDEC themselves synthesize the basement proteins laminin, collagen IV and collagen XVIII[18–20];

(d) Proliferating BDEC release fibrogenic growth factors such as epidermal growth factor (EGF), fibroblast growth factor (bFGF), transforming growth factor-β (mainly the form TGF-β2) and platelet-derived growth factor (the form PDGF-AA)[21,22];

(e) BDEC have the receptors for the epithelial mitogens EGF, leading to autocrine growth stimulation, and for hepatocyte growth factor (HGF), which is released by the surrounding rim of activated portal fibroblasts or stellate cells to be avidly internalized by proliferating BDEC[23–25].

These findings underline the close association between bile ductular proliferation and activation of the surrounding mesenchyme, a feature that is preserved in bile duct carcinomas which are characterized by a strong desmoplastic reaction. Figure 1 summarizes triggers, cells and growth factors/cytokines that are involved in fibrogenesis of PBC.

A scheme that attempts to incorporate various hypotheses regarding the yet-unsolved pathogenesis of bile duct damage in PBC is shown in Figure 2. Triggers and predisposing factors include:

(a) Enterobacterial and mycobacterial antigens[26];

(b) Self antigens like the ketoacid dehydrogenase complex, that can be presented on BDEC to initiate an immune response[27,28];

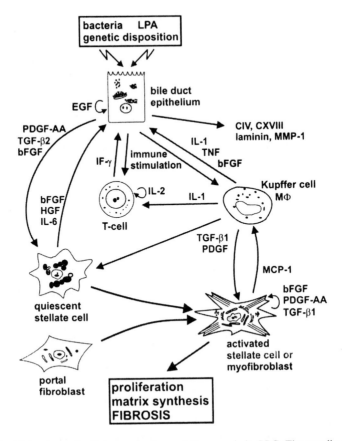

Figure 1 Molecular and cellular mechanisms of fibrogenesis in PBC. The usually quiescent portal fibroblast and the hepatic stellate cell are activated to transform into a myofibroblast-like cell that is characterized by actin stress fibers, a hypertrophied rough endoplasmic reticulum, a high rate of proliferation and an excessive ECM synthesis. Although not shown here, other cell types, such as sinusoidal endothelial cells (which are central to angiogenesis and, once damaged, secrete fibrogenic factors), activated platelets (releasing fibrogenic factors) and granulocytes (producing reactive oxygen species and thus inducing the release of cytokines in other cells), are also involved in the pathogenesis of liver fibrosis. MΦ, macrophage; LPA, lipopolysaccharide; bFGF, basic fibroblast growth factor; EGF, epidermal growth factor; HGF, hepatocyte growth factor; IF, interferon; IL, interleukin; TNF, tumor necrosis factor; TGF, transforming growth factor; PDGF, platelet-derived growth factor; MCP, macrophage chemotactic peptide; ET, endothelin.

(c) A (relatively weak) genetic association of PBC with HLA-DRw3/8[29];

(d) Additional toxic agents and mediators such as lipopolysaccharide (LPA) and tumor necrosis factor (TNF)[26].

THE HEPATIC EXTRACELLULAR MATRIX

The extracellular matrix (ECM) is not a metabolically inert material that merely serves as a framework for the functionally important parenchyma.

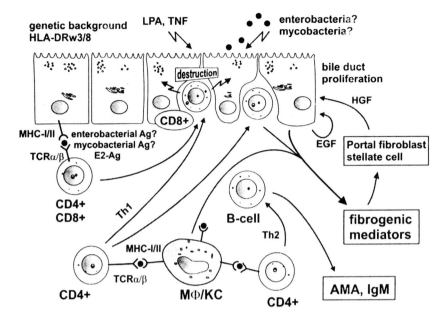

Figure 2 Suggested triggers of fibrogenesis in PBC. The simplified model illustrates how several triggers may finally lead to bile duct epithelial damage which initiates a cascade involving bile ductular proliferation and recruitment of portal fibroblasts/stellate cells which mutually interact by secretion of mediators that stimulate proliferation and fibrogenesis. AMA, antimitochondrial antibodies; E2-Ag, antigens of the ketoglutarate dehydrogenase complex; EGF, epidermal growth factor; HGF, hepatocyte growth factor; LPA, lipopolysaccharide; MΦ/KC, macrophage/Kupffer cell; TNF, tumor necrosis factor.

It may rather be defined as a complex assembly of macromolecules that rapidly undergoes remodeling after injury, in order to re-establish cellular functions and tissue homeostasis. Its macromolecules provide resident and immigrating (e.g. inflammatory) cells with signals that are necessary for proliferation, differentiation, directed migration, or for the establishment of cell polarity[8,30]. These signals are mediated by cellular receptors for ECM proteins, such as the integrins. The molecules of the ECM comprise collagens, non-collagenous glycoproteins, glycosaminoglycans, proteoglycans and elastin, including hybrids with structural and functional properties that are characteristic not only for a single class. In addition, other molecules that can specifically associate with the classical ECM components, can be considered as ECM constituents. Examples are ECM-degrading matrix metalloproteinases (MMPs) and their inhibitors (the tissue inhibitors of metalloproteinases, TIMPs)[31,32], certain crosslinking enzymes, such as lysyl hydroxylase and tissue transglutaminase, and a variety of growth factors and cytokines. Binding of growth factors by certain matrix molecules leads to their storage in a matrix-dependent pattern and to modulation of their biological activities[25,32-35]. Once released by matrix-degrading enzymes, such as the MMPs, these factors can initiate cell proliferation, angiogenesis and

ECM deposition, processes that are directed at the restitution of organ homeostasis.

SUITABLE *IN-VIVO* MODELS FOR ANTIFIBROTIC DRUG TESTING

In order to evaluate the antifibrotic potential of a drug, selection of appropriate animal models that resemble human PBC is essential. Most studies have applied models of injury that are induced by free radicals, severe necrosis or inflammation, such as fibrosis/cirrhosis due to carbon tetrachloride, dimethylnitrosamine, and pig serum[36,37]. These models do not resemble PBC. Furthermore, many drugs that act as radical scavengers, antioxidants, or antiphlogistics, prevent fibrosis in these animals but lack efficiency in man. In our hands, the best model is secondary biliary fibrosis in the rat induced by complete occlusion of the bile ducts by retrograde injection of the sclerosant sodium amidotrizoate. As in late stages of PBC, this model is characterized by proliferating bile ductules with the accompanying fibrosis, resulting in a roughly tenfold increase of liver collagen within six weeks, and by the virtual absence of necrosis and inflammation[38,39]. It therefore seems to be suited to testing for pure antifibrotic effects. However, unlike PBC, mechanical obstruction to bile flow is the trigger for ductular proliferation in this model.

POTENTIAL ANTIFIBROTIC AGENTS

There are no reliable data on the antifibrotic effect of certain drugs in patients with PBC. Therefore, this section can only give a short and subjective overview of agents that appear to have or not have some effect in experimental models or in man. Although interferons, especially interferon-γ, suppress collagen synthesis in mesenchymal cells *in vitro*, including hepatic stellate cells[40–42], their antifibrotic effect *in vivo* is less convincing. This may be due to their immune stimulatory activities on non-fibroblastic cells and lends a note of caution that final proof of an antifibrotic activity can only be obtained *in vivo*. Nonetheless, some clinical studies have shown that the aminoterminal procollagen III peptide, a surrogate serum marker of fibrogenesis, may decrease in patients treated for hepatitis B and C with interferon-2α, even when a viral response does not occur[43,44]. However, patients in these studies have not been controlled for alcohol consumption which may have fallen during interferon therapy. A recent study described an antifibrotic effect of interferon-α2b in rat secondary fibrosis after bile duct ligation[45]. Unfortunately, the author used low numbers of rats and a human interferon preparation that is thought to have little activity in the rat.

Only high doses of *prostaglandin E* are antifibrotic in rat models of liver fibrosis induced by nutrient deficiency or biliary fibrosis[46,47]. Some oral drugs with few side-effects have reappeared in therapeutic trials. Polyunsaturated lecithin (PUL), with the active agent dilinoleyl-phosphatidylcholine, prevented severe fibrosis and cirrhosis in baboons fed a diet containing 50% ethanol, probably by upregulating stellate cell collagenase activity[48].

Silymarin, a defined phytopharmacon with the polyphenole silibinin as major active compound, reduced collagen accumulation by 30% in rat secondary biliary fibrosis, an effect not reached by other agents in this model. The antifibrotic effect of silymarin was even observed when the drug was fed during the second half of the experiment when fibrosis was already established[39], whereas ursodeoxycholic acid caused a fall in serum cholestasis parameters[49] but did not inhibit collagen accumulation at concentrations of 10 and 20 mg kg^{-1} day^{-1}. Pentoxifylline could reduce liver collagen by 20% in rat secondary biliary fibrosis only when given from the beginning of the experiment[50]. Although collagen synthesis inhibitors, such as agents that block the collagen-processing enzyme prolyl 4-hydroxylase are effective *in vitro*, they are mainly taken up by hepatocytes and not by the collagen-producing mesenchymal cells. Molecular strategies are aimed at suppressing the synthesis of fibrillar collagens, mainly types I and III, which represent 80–90% of the hepatic collagen in fibrosis, at blocking extracellular collagen crosslinking which makes it less susceptible to degradation, or at activating the collagenases (Figure 3). All these steps can be inhibited *in vitro* without causing major toxicity for fibroblastic cells. However, multicellular organisms are far more complex, with interfering drugs either being inactive or too toxic, problems that mainly result from a yet-inefficient drug targeting to the key ECM-producing cells, namely the activated hepatic stellate cell and the activated portal fibroblast.

Novel targeted approaches are based on the neutralization or localized removal of fibrogenic growth factors. Thus, in a rat model of glomerular fibrosis, the fibrogenic activity of TGF-β1, a mediator that can enhance ECM deposition and inhibit collagenase expression, can be blocked by intramuscular injection of the gene encoding decorin, a small matrix proteoglycan that binds and sequesters TGF-β1 in the ECM[51]. Similarly, PDGF, a potent mitogen for hepatic stellate cells[52], is bound to liver collagens at sites of excessive release[53]. Since this interaction is mediated by a single acidic sequence present in the collagens, peptide analogs can be designed that remove the excess of PDGF deposited in the ECM. A promising target is induction of a so-called 'stress relaxation' of the fibrogenic cells. Stress relaxation occurs once mesenchymal cells are placed from a 'stressed' two-dimensional environment, mimicking a situation of wounding, into a relaxed three-dimensional environment, inducing quiescence[54]. It reverses the fibrogenic cellular phenotype, leads to a decrease in collagen synthesis, an increase in collagenase activity, and it mitigates or even abrogates signals transferred via the receptors for PDGF and other mitogenic growth factors[55] (Figure 4). A stress signal is also transmitted to fibroblastic cells by nanomolar amounts of soluble collagen VI which is rapidly released from the ECM during remodeling and may act as an auto- and paracrine growth factor[56]. Since the collagen VI-induced stress and growth response depends on receptor clustering, collagen VI-derived peptides could be used to induce stress relaxation and thus a non-fibrogenic cellular phenotype.

SERUM MARKERS FOR LIVER FIBROSIS

Suitable serum assays for liver fibrosis should fulfil the following requirements: They ought to:

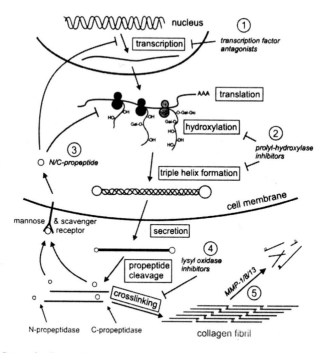

Figure 3 Steps of collagen biosynthesis. The scheme applies to the well-studied fibril-forming collagens. Collagen mRNA is transcribed from the gene and translated into protein in the rough endoplasmic reticulum. During translation, the nascent polypeptide chains are hydroxyl-ated on lysine and proline residues, glycosylated and assembled to the triple helix, starting from the C-terminal end. After secretion, N- and C-terminal propeptides are cleaved off by specific proteases and fibril growth occurs by quarter-staggered lateral assembly. Fibrils are then stabilized by formation of covalent crosslinks. Antifibrotic approaches could target either collagen biosynthesis (① blocking collagen gene specific transcription factors; ② inhibition of the production of thermodynamically stable triple helical collagen by blocking the enzyme prolyl hydroxylase; ③ inhibition of collagen gene transcription and collagen mRNA translation by procollagen peptides that are cleaved by extracellular propeptidases, and which can be taken up by the cell to serve as feed-back inhibitors), ④ stabilization of the extracellular collagen fibrils by crosslinking with the matrix-bound enzyme lysyl hydroxylase, or ⑤ activation of collagenases. Modified from Reference 30.

(a) Be specific for the liver, with no major contribution by other organs;

(b) Be sensitive to detect minor changes of fibrogenesis and fibrolysis;

(c) Reflect either fibrogenesis, fibrolysis or the amount of connective tissue deposited in the liver;

(d) Have a known biological half-life and known major routes of disposal and excretion, thus allowing a better interpretation of changing serum levels in patients with reduced kidney or liver function;

(e) Derive from a defined cellular source in the diseased liver (mainly the activated mesenchymal cells) in order to exclude interference by a func-tionally and synthetically compromised parenchyma;

(f) Be measurable by sensitive, rapid and easy-to-perform assay formats, such as the ELISA technique, obviating expensive equipment or a

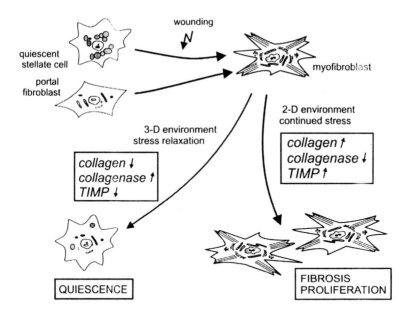

Figure 4 Stress relaxation and induction of cellular quiescence. Continued mechanical stress triggers and maintains the fibrogenic phenotype. The fibrogenic phenotype is characterized by a responsive (stressed) conformation of certain ECM receptors, such as the integrins $\alpha 1\beta 1$, $\alpha 2\beta 1$ and $\alpha 5\beta 1$ that serve as ECM-directed environmental sensors. Furthermore, it may be accompanied by an enhanced expression and responsiveness of the cellular receptors for fibrogenic growth factors such as TGF-β, bFGF and PDGF. Independently of growth factors, stressed integrins can enhance the expression of collagens and the tissue inhibitor of metallo-proteinases (TIMP-1), and downregulate collagenase (MMP-1). This program is aimed at rapid wound closure, is usually self-limited and subsides once the wound is filled with an appropriate ECM. However, it remains continuously operative in active liver fibrosis. Novel therapies can be designed that utilize so-called adhesive recognition sequences from ECM molecules to compete with the ECM receptors, inducing a relaxed mesenchymal phenotype, with subsequent upregulation of collagenases and downregulation of collagens and TIMPs.

nuclear medicine department;
(g) Be standardized and validated by reference laboratories to ensure comparability of results.

Presently, the available serum markers for liver fibrosis do not meet the requirements of ideal parameters (reviewed in References 57–61), although biochemical, animal experimental and clinical studies have provided some information that permits a preliminary judgement of how far certain markers might mirror fibrogenesis and/or fibrolysis in the liver. Thus, most of the measurable connective tissue antigens show the highest levels in active liver diseases, with only minor contributions by other systemic inflammatory or fibrotic conditions, such as pulmonary fibrosis, rheumatoid arthritis and the so-called 'collagen diseases'. When selecting assays for liver fibrosis, one has to consider the source and distribution of the target antigen. Thus, collagen/procollagen I, the major ECM protein of liver, is also the main structural protein of bone, making its various assays unsuitable for the

Table 1 Serum assays for liver fibrosis

	Fibrogenesis	Fibrolysis	Liver specificity
PIIINP	+	(+) (acute)	+
PIIICP	+	−	+
PIVCP	− (?)	+	+
PIVNP	− (?)	+	+
Collagen VI	+	+ (mesenchymal stress)	(+)
Undulin	−	+ (portal)	+
Tenascin	+ (lobular)	−	(+)
Laminin	+ (?)	+ (?)	(+)
Hyaluronan	+ (?)	+ (?)	(+)
TIMP-1	+	−	+ (?)
MMP-1	−	+	+ (?)
MMP-2	+ (?)	− (?)	(+)

PIIINP, N-terminal propeptide of procollagen III; PIIINP may also reflect fibrolysis in acute bouts of hepatitis. PIIICP, C-terminal propeptide of procollagen III; this assay has recently been developed and appears to reflect only fibrogenesis. PIVCP, C-terminal propeptide of procollagen IV (NC1-fragment). PIVNP, N-terminal propeptide of procollagen IV (7-S collagen). TIMP-1, tissue inhibitor of metalloproteinases 1. MMP-1, matrix metalloproteinase 1 (interstitial collagenase). MMP-2, basement membrane collagenase; elevated levels of this enzyme may reflect unfortunate remodeling of the liver. Liver specificity denotes that highest levels are observed in liver diseases. Markers in bold are considered most useful to assess ECM metabolism in liver disease

monitoring of fibrogenic liver diseases. Another problem is the heterogeneity of circulating antigens usually encountered, requiring a clear characterization of the proteins or fragments which are detected by a given assay. A well-known example is the aminoterminal propeptide of procollagen III (PIIINP). PIIINP immunoreactivity in serum elutes as four major fractions: the intact aminopropeptide of Mr 50 kDa, a prominent fraction of its degradation product, fragment Col 1 of Mr 10 kDa, and two fractions of higher Mr, probably representing dimeric propeptide and propeptide linked to the collagen helix. In acute liver disease, the proportion of the intact propeptide of Mr 50 kDa may increase relative to the other fractions. Only intact PIIINP that is released in stoichiometric amounts when newly secreted procollagen III is incorporated into the growing collagen fibril can be attributed to fibrogenesis.

Reports of the value of PIIINP as an independent parameter predicting prognosis or fibrogenesis in PBC range from enthusiastic[62-64] to disappointing[65]. This may, in part, relate to the low sensitivity of PIIINP and many other serum fibrosis markers to detect early stages of the disease and subtle differences in collagen turnover, or to variant assay versions that were marketed during recent years. Table 1 lists some of the serum fibrosis markers that may be useful in future studies of antifibrotic drug effects in PBC. It must be kept in mind that these markers still await validation in large prospective follow-up studies of patients with liver diseases and of controls. A study that will involve 500 patients with biopsies taken at the beginning and after 18–24 months, incorporating an improved histological method to quantitate fibrosis as well as a broad spectrum of fibrosis markers in a 3-month interval, is currently underway on a European level. In addition, collagen synthesis and protease expression can now be quantified from fractions of diagnostic biopsies, allowing a direct correlation with the concurrently measured serum markers.

Therefore, the stage is set to attack fibrogenesis in PBC. Trials should include well-defined methods to assess histological progression of fibrosis and a selected spectrum of serum fibrosis markers. Some of these markers may soon be validated and prove useful in predicting fibrogenesis or fibrolysis, thus enabling us to predict an antifibrotic effect in an individual patient within a few weeks.

References

1. Metcalfe JV, Mitchison HC, Palmer JM, Jones DE, Bassendine MF, James OFW. Natural history of early primary biliary cirrhosis. Lancet 1996;348:1399–402.
2. Mahl T, Shockcor W, Boyer JL. Primary biliary cirrhosis; survival of a large cohort of symptomatic and asymptomatic patients followed for 24 years. J Hepatol 1994;20:707–13.
3. Locke III GR, Therneau TM, Ludwig J, Dickson ER, Lindor KD. Time course and histological progression in primary biliary cirrhosis. Hepatology 1996;23:52–6.
4. McClain C, Hill D, Schmidt J, Diehl AM. Cytokines and alcoholic liver disease. Semin Liver Dis 1993;13:170–81.
5. Gressner AM. Hepatic fibrogenesis: the puzzle of interacting cells, fibrogenic cytokines, regulatory loops, and extracellular matrix molecules. Z Gastroenterol 1992;30(S1):5–16.
6. Friedman SL. The cellular basis of hepatic fibrosis. N Engl J Med 1993;328:1826–35.
7. Adachi Y, Bradford BA, Bojes HK, Thurman RG. Inactivation of Kupffer cells prevents early alcohol-induced liver injury. Hepatology 1994;20:453–60.
8. Schuppan D, Herbst H, Milani S. Matrix, matrix synthesis and molecular networks. In: Zern MA, Reid LM, eds. Extracellular Matrix: Chemistry, Biology and Pathobiology with Emphasis on the Liver. New York: Marcel Dekker; 1993:201–54.
9. Gressner AM, Schuppan D. Cellular and molecular pathobiology, pharmacological intervention, and biochemical assessment of liver fibrosis. In: Oxford Textbook of Clinical Hepatology, 2nd edn. 1998, in press.
10. Ramadori G. The stellate cell (Ito-cell, fat-storing cell, lipocyte, perisinusoidal cell) of the liver. New insights into pathophysiology of an intriguing cell. Virchows Arch B 1991;61:147–58.
11. Pinzani M. Hepatic stellate (Ito) cells: expanding roles for a liver-specific pericyte. J Hepatol 1995;22:700–6.
12. Floege J, Eng E, Young BA, Johnson RJ. Factors involved in the regulation of mesangial cell proliferation in vitro and in vivo. Kidney Int 1993;43(S39):S47–S54.
13. Matthes H, Herbst H, Schuppan D, et al. Cellular localization of procollagen gene transcripts in inflammatory bowel diseases. Gastroenterology 1992;102:431–42.
14. Kovacs EJ, DiPietro LA. Fibrogenic cytokines and connective tissue production. FASEB J 1994;8:854–61.
15. Ross R. The pathogenesis of atherosclerosis: a perspective for the 1990's. Nature 1993;362:801–9.
16. Tuchweber B, Desmouliere A, Bochaton-Piallat LL, Rubbia-Brandt L, Gabbiani G. Proliferation and phenotypic modulation of portal fibroblasts in the early stages of cholestatic fibrosis in the rat. Lab Invest 1996;74:265–78.
17. Milani S, Herbst H, Schuppan D, Riecken EO, Stein H. Procollagen expression by nonparenchymal rat liver cells in experimental biliary fibrosis. Gastroenterology 1990;98:175–84.
18. Milani S, Herbst H, Schuppan D, Surrenti C, Riecken EO, Stein H. Cellular localization of type I, III and IV procollagen gene transcripts in normal and fibrotic human liver. Am J Pathol 1990;137:59–70.
19. Milani S, Herbst H, Schuppan D, Riecken EO, Stein H. Cellular localization of laminin gene transcripts in normal and fibrotic human liver. Am J Pathol 1989;134:1175–82.
20. Cramer T, Bauer M, Herbst H, Riecken EO, Schuppan D. Hepatocytes are the major source of collagen type XVIII in human liver. J Hepatol 1997;26(S1):A132(abstract).

21. Milani S, Herbst H, Schuppan D, Stein H, Surrenti C. Transforming growth factors $\beta 1$ and $\beta 2$ are differentially expressed in fibrotic liver disease. Am J Pathol 1991;139:1221–9.
22. Perez Napoli J, Prentice D, Niinami C, Bishop GA, Desmond P, McCaugham GW. Sequential increases in the intrahepatic expression of epidermal growth factor, basic fibroblast growth factor, and transforming growth factor β in a bile duct ligated rat model of cirrhosis. Hepatology 1997;26:624–33.
23. Matsumoto K, Fuji H, Michalopoulos G, Fung JJ, Demetris AJ. Human biliary epithelial cells secrete and respond to cytokines and hepatocyte growth factor in vitro: interleukin-6, hepatocyte growth factor, and epidermal growth factor promote DANN synthesis in vitro. Hepatology 1994;20:376–82.
24. Joplin R, Hishida T, Tsubouchi H, et al. Human intrahepatic biliary epithelial cells proliferate in vitro in response to human hepatocyte growth factor. J Clin Invest 1992;90:1284–90.
25. Schuppan D, Schmid M, Somasundaram R, et al. Collagens retain hepatocyte growth factor (HGF) in the liver extracellular matrix. Gastroenterology 1998;114:139–52.
26. Hopf U, Mller B, Stemerowicz R, et al. Escherichia coli rough R mutants in the gut and lipid A in the liver from patients with primary biliary cirrhosis (PBC). Lancet 1989; 2:1419–22.
27. Sundin U, Sundqvist KG. Plasma membrane association of primary biliary cirrhosis mitochondrial marker antigen M2. Clin Exp Immunol 1991;83:407–12.
28. Joplin R, Lindsay JG, Johnson J, Strain A, Neuberger J. Membrane dihydrolipoamide acetyltransferase (E2) on human biliary epithelial cells in primary biliary cirrhosis. Lancet 1992;339:93–4.
29. Manns MP, Bremm A, Schneider PM, et al. HLA DRw8 and complement C4 deficiency as risk factors in primary biliary cirrhosis. Gastroenterology 1991;101:1367–73.
30. Schuppan D, Gressner AM. Function and metabolism of collagens and other extracellular matrix proteins. In: Oxford Textbook of Clinical Hepatology, 2nd edn. 1998, in press.
31. Birkedahl-Hansen H. Proteolytic remodeling of the extracellular matrix. Curr Opin Cell Biol 1995;7:728–35.
32. Arthur MJP. Collagenases and liver fibrosis. J Hepatol 1995;22:43–8.
33. Nathan C, Sporn M. Cytokines in context. J Cell Biol 1991;113:981–6.
34. Ruoslahti E, Yamaguchi Y. Proteoglycans as modulators of growth factor activities. Cell 1991;64:867–9.
35. Schuppan D, Somasundaram R, Dieterich W, Ehnis T, Bauer M. The extracellular matrix in cellular differentiation and proliferation. Ann NY Acad Sci 1994;733:87–102.
36. Tamayo R. Is cirrhosis of the liver experimentally produced by CCl_4 an adequate model of human cirrhosis? Hepatology 1984;3:112–20.
37. Tsukamoto H, Matsuoka M, French SW. Experimental models of hepatic fibrosis: an overview. Semin Liver Dis 1990;10:56–65.
38. Gerling B, Becker M, Waldschmidt J, Schuppan D. Elevated serum aminoterminal procollagen-III-peptide parallels collagen accumulation in rats with secondary biliary fibrosis. J Hepatol 1996;25:79–84.
39. Boigk G, Stroedter L, Herbst H, Waldschmidt, Riecken EO, Schuppan D. Silymarin retards hepatic collagen accumulation in early and advanced biliary fibrosis secondary to bile duct obliteration in the rat. Hepatology 1997;26:643–49.
40. Rosenbloom J, Feldman G, Freundlich G, Jimenez SA. Transcriptional control of human diploid fibroblast collagen synthesis by interferon. Biochem Biophys Res Commun 1984;123:365–72.
41. Rockey DC, Maher JJ, Jarnagin WR, Gabbiani G, Friedman SL. Inhibition of rat lipocyte activation in culture by interferon-γ. Hepatology 1992;16:776–84.
42. Mallat A, Preaux AM, Blazejewski S, Rosenbaum J, Dhumeaux D, Mavier P. Interferon alfa and gamma inhibit proliferation and collagen synthesis of human Ito cells in culture. Hepatology 1995;21:1003–10.
43. Camps J, Castilla A, Ruiz J, Civeira MP, Prieto J. Randomised trial of lymphoblastoid α-interferon in chronic hepatitis C. Effects on inflammation, fibrogenesis and viremia. J Hepatol 1993;17:390–96.
44. Suou T, Hosho K, Kishimoto Y, Horie Y, Kawasaki H. Long-term decrease in serum N-terminal propeptide of type III procollagen in patients with chronic hepatitis C treated with interferon alfa. Hepatology 1995;22:426–31.

45. Muriel P. Alpha interferon prevents liver collagen deposition and damage induced by prolonged bile duct obstruction in the rat. J Hepatol 1996;24:614–21.
46. Ruwart MJ, Rush BD, Snyder KF, et al. 16,16-Dimethyl prostaglandin E2 delays collagen formation in nutritional injury in rat liver. Hepatology 1988;8:61–4.
47. Beno DWA, Espinal R, Edelstein BM, Davis BH. Administration of prostaglandin E1 analog reduces rat hepatic and Ito cell collagen gene expression and accumulation after bile duct ligation injury. Hepatology 1993;17:707–14.
48. Lieber CS, Robins SJ, Li J, et al. Phosphatidylcholine protects against fibrosis and cirrhosis in the baboon. Gastroenterology 1994;106:152–9.
49. Boigk G, Stroedter L, Herbst H, Waldschmidt J, Riecken EO, Schuppan D. Ursodeoxycholic acid ameliorates parameters of cholestasis, but does not prevent collagen accumulation in rat secondary biliary fibrosis. Gastroenterology 1997;112:A372(abstract).
50. Raetsch C, Boigk G, Stroedter L, et al. Pentoxifylline inhibits hepatic collagen deposition in early but not advanced rat biliary fibrosis. Gastroenterology 1996;110:A1301(abstract).
51. Isaka Y, Brees DK, Ikegaya K, et al. Gene therapy by skeletal muscle expression of decorin prevents fibrotic disease in rat kidney. Nature Med 1996;2:418–23.
52. Pinzani M, Gesualdo L, Sabbah GM, Abboud HE. Effects of platelet-derived growth factor and other mitogens on DNA synthesis and growth of cultured rat liver fat storing cells. J Clin Invest 1989;84:1786–94.
53. Somasundaram R, Schuppan D. Platelet derived growth factor (PDGF AA, AB and BB) binds to collagens type I-VI: evidence for common collagenous epitopes. J Biol Chem 1996;271:26884–91.
54. Grinnell F. Fibroblasts, myofibroblasts and wound contraction. J Cell Biol 1994;124:401–4.
55. Lin YC, Grinnell F. Decreased level of PDGF-stimulated receptor autophosphorylation by fibroblasts in mechanically relaxed collagen matrices. J Cell Biol 1993;122:663–72.
56. Atkinson J, Ruehl M, Becker J, Ackermann R, Schuppan D. Collagen VI regulates normal and transformed mesenchymal cell proliferation in vitro. Exp Cell Res 1996;228:283–91.
57. Risteli L, Risteli J. Noninvasive methods for detection of of organ fibrosis. In: Rojkind M, ed. Focus on Connective Tissue in Health and Disease. Boca Raton: CRC Press; 1990:61–98.
58. Plebani M, Burlina A. Biochemical markers of hepatic fibrosis. Clin Biochem 1991; 24:219–39.
59. Schuppan D, Stölzel U, Oesterling C, Somasundaram R. Serum assays for liver fibrosis. J Hepatol 1995;22(Suppl. 2):82–8.
60. Schuppan D, Aksü T, Libuda P, Koszka C, Herbst H. Serum markers for liver fibrosis – current and future developments. In: Reichen J, Poupon R, eds. Surrogate markers to assess efficacy of treatment in chronic liver diseases. Dordrecht: Kluwer; 1996:105–22.
61. Schuppan D, Jia JD, Boigk G, Oesterling C. Liver fibrogenesis – therapy and non-invasive assessment. In: Galmiche JP, Gournay J, eds. Recent Advances in the Pathophysiology of Gastrointestinal and Liver Diseases. Paris: John Libbey; 1997:243–57.
62. Savolainen ER, Miettinen TA, Pikkarainen P, Salaspuro MP, Kivirikko KI. Enzymes of collagen synthesis and type III procollagen aminopropeptide in the evaluation of D-penicillamine and medroxyprogesterone treatments in primary biliary cirrhosis. Gut 1983; 24:136–42.
63. Niemelä O, Risteli L, Sotaniemi EA, Stenback F, Risteli J. Serum basement membrane and type III procollagen related antigens in primary biliary cirrhosis. J Hepatol 1988;6:307–14.
64. Babbs C, Smith A, Hunt LP, Rowan BP, Habouchi NY, Warnes TW. Type III procollagen peptide: a marker of disease activity and prognosis in primary biliary cirrhosis. Lancet 1988;2:1021–4.
65. Beukers R, van Zanten RAA, Schalm SW. Serial determination of type III procollagen amino propeptide serum levels in patients with histologically progressive and non-progressive primary biliary cirrhosis. J Hepatol 1992;14:22–9.

9
Natural history models of primary biliary cirrhosis

W. R. KIM AND E. R. DICKSON

INTRODUCTION

The natural progression of primary biliary cirrhosis (PBC) has been modeled by a number of investigators based on Cox's proportional hazards analysis[1-3]. The utility of these models is largely two-fold. On the one hand, these models have been used as a clinical tool in assessing prognosis with or without treatment. For example, the natural history model for PBC has been used in determining prognosis following transplantation, thereby assisting transplant physicians and surgeons in their decisions about patient selection and timing of transplantation[4]. On the other hand, these models are useful from the standpoint of clinical research. For instance, the prognostic indices of the models may be used as parameters of disease severity in risk stratification in clinical trials evaluating new treatment modalities[5].

In this review on prognostic models of primary biliary cirrhosis, the development, validation, and application of the Mayo natural history model for PBC are presented. We also discuss some of the caveats to be exercised in the use of this model. Finally, we review the application of the model in patients being treated with ursodeoxycholic acid.

NATURAL HISTORY MODELS FOR PRIMARY BILIARY CIRRHOSIS

Survival models of PBC based on Cox's proportional hazards assumptions incorporate clinical and biochemical variables to compute a summary index of disease severity, which, in turn, may be used in an equation to arrive at survival prediction. The clinical variables identified in these models as independent predictors of survival are summarized in Table 1. Of these, the prognostic model developed by investigators at the Mayo Clinic has undergone rigorous validation and been used most widely, at least in North America.

Table 1 Independent predictors of survival in PBC

Mayo[1]	Yale[2]	European[3]
Age	Age	Age
Bilirubin	Bilirubin	Bilirubin
Albumin	Hepatomegaly	Albumin
Prothrombin time	Fibrosis/cirrhosis	Cirrhosis
Edema		Cholestasis

Table 2 Computational formula for the risk score for PBC and PSC

$$
\begin{aligned}
R = {} & 0.04 \ (\text{age}) \\
& + 0.87 \log_e (\text{bilirubin}) \\
& - 2.53 \log_e (\text{albumin}) \\
& + 2.38 \log_e (\text{prothrombin time}) \\
& + 0.86 \ (\text{edema*})
\end{aligned}
$$

*0 = no edema without diuretic therapy; 0.5 = edema without diuretic therapy or edema resolved with diuretic therapy; 1 = edema despite diuretic therapy.

The Mayo model for PBC was developed based on 312 patients who had been carefully diagnosed and enrolled in clinical trials for D-penicillamine[1]. As this medication was found not to provide therapeutic benefits and the study protocol stipulated that patients should not take any other medications which may potentially influence the clinical course of the disease, the progression of disease in this group of patients was deemed appropriate to represent the natural history of PBC.

Of the 312 patients, 125 died after a median follow-up of 66 months. Nineteen underwent liver transplantation, while 160 were alive and being followed. A number of demographic, clinical, biochemical and histologic variables in these patients were examined, of which five were identified as statistically and clinically significant predictors of survival. These include the patient's age, presence or absence of peripheral edema, prothrombin time and the serum levels of albumin and bilirubin. Based on these variables, a summary score, or risk score (R), was obtained and patient survival was estimated (Table 2).

This model has been validated using a number of different data sets. Initially, the model was applied to 106 patients with PBC at the Mayo Clinic who were not included in the treatment trial. Subsequently, extramural validation was undertaken using data on 176 patients from two institutions outside the Mayo Clinic[6]. On both occasions, the Mayo model was able to predict the actual survival accurately. Although there had been other models published previously, the Mayo model gained most popularity for two reasons: the advantage of not requiring liver histology and the rigorous validation to which the model was subject.

NUMERIC EXAMPLES

Although the derivation of the survival model with the inherent intricacies of survival statistics may appear complex by the uninitiated, the actual

Table 3 Underlying survival function for the Mayo models for PBC $\{S(t) = S_0(t)^{\exp(R - 5.07)}\}$

t (years)	0	1	2	3	4	5	6	7
Original (time to death)	1	0.970	0.941	0.883	0.833	0.774	0.721	0.651

application of the model is relatively straightforward. The expected survival is derived using two steps: First, a risk score is computed according to the formula. Then, by feeding the risk score as the exponent in the equation $\{S(t) = S_0(t)^{\exp(R - R_0)}\}$, the survival probability at each year up to seven years may be computed. All of these computations can be readily performed on a programmable hand-held calculator or a personal computer.

Consider a hypothetical patient with PBC and the following variables: age = 55 years, serum total bilirubin = 4.0 mg/dl, serum albumin = 3.0 g/dl, prothrombin time = 13 s, and peripheral edema which was resolved with diuretic treatment. The risk score for this PBC patient is computed by: $R = 0.04$ (age) $+ 0.87 \log$ (bilirubin) $- 2.53 \log$ (albumin) $+ 2.38 \log$ (prothrombin time) $+ 0.86$ (edema) $= 0.04(55) + 0.87 \log(4.0) - 2.53 \log(3.0) + 2.38 \log(13) + 0.86(0.5) = 7.11$. From $S(t) = S_0(t)^{\exp(R - R_0)}$ where R_0 is a constant (5.07 for PBC), $S(t)$ or probability of survival at time t is a constant $S_0(t)$ raised to the power of $e^{(R - R_0)}$. For example, to compute the estimated 1- and 5-year survival in this patient, $S_0(1) = 0.970$ and $S_0(5) = 0.774$ are taken from Table 3(a). Inserting an R of 7.11 into the equation $S(t) = S_0(t)^{\exp(R - R_0)}$, we get $S(1) = 0.970^{\exp(7.11 - 5.07)} = 0.79$ and $S(5) = 0.774^{\exp(7.11 - 5.07)} = 0.14$. Thus, this patient who has a risk score of 7.11 has a 79% chance of surviving the next year and a 14% chance of surviving the next 5 years (Figure 1).

We have recently developed software to implement our PBC natural history model in a user-friendly manner. The software is in a hypertext document, a format used in the World Wide Web, as shown in Figure 2. In this figure, computation of the above numeric example is being displayed using this software. The age, bilirubin, albumin, and prothrombin time are entered. For the edema variables, appropriate buttons are pushed. Upon a click of the Compute button, the risk score is calculated and survival estimates shown in the table. Interested readers are encouraged to contact the authors for a copy of the software.

CAVEATS

We would like to remind the reader of a few caveats in using the Mayo natural history model. First, the model was derived based on albumin levels obtained by electrophoresis. Most clinical laboratories employ colorimetric methods for measurement of serum albumin concentrations, which tend to overestimate the albumin level. Although the difference between the two techniques is usually small and its impact on the risk score minor, the user must be aware of such. A similar caution may be applied to the laboratory methodology determining the prothrombin time. Prothrombin time is dependent on the thromboplastin reagent used in the laboratory. A recent report

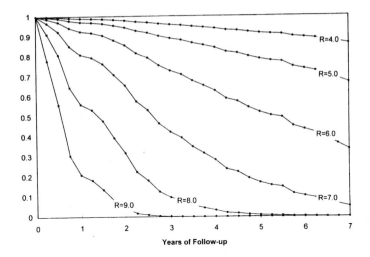

Figure 1 Survival estimates as predicted by the Mayo natural history model for primary biliary cirrhosis according to risk score.

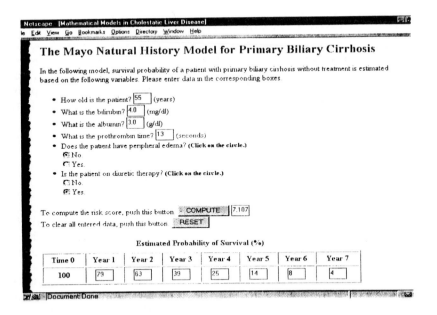

Figure 2 Illustration of computer software to compute the Mayo natural history model. This example shows Netscape Navigator version 3.0. Microsoft Internet Explorer may also be used to run this software. When all necessary data are entered and the Compute button pressed, the risk score and survival estimates are returned instantaneously.

suggested that the variability of prothrombin time cannot be overcome by using the international normalized ratio (INR) in patients with chronic liver disease. Instead, prothrombin time activity percentage (% dilution of normal sample with an equivalent prothrombin time) appears to minimize variation in prothrombin time measurement in patients with hepatic failure[7].

Second, care must be taken not to extrapolate the model outside the range within which the model was created and validated[8]. In the orginal model, the risk score in the majority of patients (80%) ranged between 4.03 and 7.67. In the validation set, the range of the risk score for the middle 80% was 4.24–7.45. The accuracy of survival estimates as predicted by the model may be less reliable when the risk score is very high or very low.

Third, when the model is applied in more recent data sets, an adjustment may be necessary to account for the fact that the original model was developed based on a data set in which liver transplantation was infrequent. In the last decade or so, survival of liver transplant recipients, particularly those with cholestatic disease, has been greatly improved[4,9]. Partly because of these good results, liver transplantation is being performed as an elective procedure before patients approach the terminal phase of disease progression. It is likely that there has been an increasing gap between the time patients would have died without transplantation and the time they actually undergo transplantation[9].

These developments present an issue in applying the natural history model to compare the model's prediction and actual patient survival data in a group of patients. For example, if all liver transplants in the data set are considered as failure, i.e. treated the same as deaths, an overly pessimistic estimate will result, as many patients undergoing transplantation would have lived for a significant length of time without a transplant. On the other hand, if liver transplants are ignored and only deaths are considered as end points, a bias to the contrary is produced. In such case, liver transplant recipients are being considered the same as those who do not require transplants.

NATURAL HISTORY MODEL IN THE ERA OF URSODEOXYCHOLIC ACID

Recently, ursodeoxycholic acid (UDCA) has been established as an effective treatment for PBC. UDCA influences several aspects of liver disease in patients with PBC. All trials have consistently shown that UDCA effectively lowers serum bilirubin levels[5,10] Other biochemical parameters, such as serum alkaline phosphatase and aminotransferases, also improve although markers of hepatic synthetic function may not show significant changes. In addition, UDCA prolongs survival and delays the need for liver transplantation[11]. A recent analysis on 533 patients from pooled data based on the three largest trials for UDCA showed that survival is significantly improved by UDCA therapy[12].

In light of these effects of UDCA therapy in PBC patients and the fact that serum bilirubin is the most influential variable in the determination of the risk score in the natural history model, questions have been raised as to

Table 4 Observed versus expected events as predicted by the natural history model at entry and after 6 months of ursodeoxycholic acid therapy

	At entry			At 6 months		
Risk score	n	Observed	Expected	n	Observed	Expected
< 4.50	41	2	3.9	53	2	3.6
4.50–5.37	21	1	5.8	16	2	3.6
5.37–6.42	16	6	9.4	11	6	5.4
> 6.42	10	7	14.3	5	4	3.2
Overall	88	16	33.3	85	14	15.8

whether the Mayo natural history model is still applicable in patients receiving UDCA. In other words, does the decrease in the risk score attendant to the lowered bilirubin from UDCA administration match the reduction in the risk of death?

Kilmurry *et al.* applied the Mayo natural history model in 222 patients with PBC who enrolled in the Canadian randomized controlled trial of UDCA[13]. One hundred and eleven patients received UDCA and 111 received placebo. Following completion of the study period of 24 months, more thn half the study subjects in both groups were continued or started on UDCA. Patients were followed for a mean of 4.0 years. Each patient's risk score was computed at entry and after 6 months of treatment. Patients were classified into three categories according to the risk score: the low-risk group was defined by a risk score of less than 5.37; the intermediate-risk group by a risk score between 5.37 and 6.42; and the high-risk group by a risk score greater than 6.42. Survival of patients in the treatment and placebo groups was analyzed considering liver transplantation as well as death as failure.

In the placebo group, the Mayo risk score either at entry or at 6 months correctly classified patients with statistically distinct survival, as expected. In the UDCA-treatment group, low-, intermediate-, and high-risk groups determined at entry and 6 months had statistically significantly different survival. The authors concluded that although UDCA has a definite effect on serum bilirubin levels, the effect does not eliminate the predictive power of the Mayo natural history model.

A similar analysis was undertaken based on data accumulated at the Mayo Clinic[14]. This analysis focused on 89 patients who constituted the treatment arm in a randomized controlled trial for UDCA. These patients were followed for a median of 4.6 years while on UDCA. Table 4 compares the utility of the Mayo risk score as calculated at entry and after 6 months of treatment. When the model was applied using data at entry, patients on UDCA therapy had approximately one half as many deaths or transplants as the Mayo model would have predicted based on the pretreatment data. In contrast, when the model was recalculated using data after 6 months of treatment, the model's prediction closely matched the actual occurrence of events.

In summary, the Mayo natural history model appears to accommodate the effects of UDCA therapy on the serum bilirubin level and the time until death or liver transplantation. When the biochemical parameters stabilize some time after the institution of UDCA, e.g. 6 months, the model can be recalculated to provide a more accurate survival estimate.

CONCLUSIONS

In the preceding sections, we have presented our natural history model for PBC and ways in which it may be used as a clinical and research tool. We also discussed evidence to support that our natural history model may still be useful in patients with ursodexoycholic acid. To the extent that all of these models are only numerical representations of real life events, users must be aware of a number of limitations which have been discussed. Moreover, no matter how sophisticated a system may be designed to refine the predictability of these models, such a model will always require human interpretation to be informative and useful. The utility of these models is maximized when they are used as an aid in decision making based on sound clinical judgement.

Acknowledgements

This work was supported by a grant (DK 34238) from the National Institutes of Health.

References

1. Dickson ER, Grambsch PM, Fleming TR, Fisher LD, Langworthy A. Prognosis in primary biliary cirrhosis: model for decision making. Hepatology 1989;10:1–7.
2. Roll J, Boyer JL, Barry D, Klatskin G. The prognostic importance of clinical and histologic features in asymptotic and symptomatic primary biliary cirrhosis. N Engl J Med 1983; 308:1–7.
3. Christensen E, Neuberger J, Crowe J, et al. Beneficial effect of azathioprine and prediction of prognosis in primary biliary cirrhosis: final result of an international trial. Gastroenterology 1985;89:1084–91.
4. Wiesner RH, Porayko MK, Dickson ER, et al. Selection and timing of liver transplantation in primary biliary cirrhosis and primary sclerosing cholangitis. Hepatology 1992;16:1290–9.
5. Lindor KD, Dickson ER, Baldus WP, et al. Ursodeoxycholic acid in the treatment of primary biliary cirrhosis. Gastroenterology 1994;106:1284–90.
6. Grambsch PM, Dickson ER, Kaplan M, LeSage G, Fleming TR, Langworthy AL. Extramural cross-validation of the Mayo primary biliary cirrhosis survival model establishes its generalizability. Hepatology 1989;10:846–50.
7. Robert A, Chazouilleres O. Prothrombin time in liver failure: time, ratio, activity percentage, or international normalized ratio? Hepatology 1996;24:1392–4.
8. Grambsch PM, Dickson ER, Wiesner RH, Langworthy A. Application of the Mayo primary biliary cirrhosis survival model to Mayo liver transplant patients. Mayo Clin Proc 1989;64:699–704.
9. Kim WR, Wiesner RH, Therneau TM, et al. Optimal timing of liver transplantation for primary biliary cirrhosis. Hepatology (In press).
10. Poupon RE, Poupon R, Balkau B. Ursodiol for the long-term treatment of primary biliary cirrhosis. N Engl J Med 1994;330:1342–7.
11. Lindor KD, Therneau TM, Jorgensen RA, Malinchoc M, Dickson ER. Effects of ursode-oxycholic acid on survival in patients with primary biliary cirrhosis. Gastroenterology 1996;110:1515–19.

12. Heathcote EJ, Lindor KD, Poupon R, *et al.* Combined analysis of randomized controlled trials of ursodeoxycholic acid in primary biliary cirrhosis. Gastroenterology 1997; 113:884–90.
13. Kilmurry MR, Heathcote EJ, Cauch-Dudek K, *et al.* Is the Mayo model for predicting survival useful after the introduction of ursodeoxycholic acid treatment for primary biliary cirrhosis? Hepatology 1996;23:1148–53.
14. Lindor KD, Therneau TM, Hermans JE, Dickson ER. Mayo risk score accurately predicts patient outcome with ursodeoxycholic acid treatment of primary biliary cirrhosis [abstract]. Hepatology 1996;24:167A.

Section II
Management of primary biliary cirrhosis

10
Portal hypertension in patients with primary biliary cirrhosis

P. M. HUET, J. HUET AND J. DESLAURIERS

Primary biliary cirrhosis (PBC) is a chronic liver disease that slowly progresses over time to a true cirrhosis when regenerating nodules are found on liver biopsies (stage IV according to Ludwig's criteria). Portal hypertension should then occur with the development of esophageal and gastric varices that, when of a large size, may bleed.

There is a paucity of studies on portal hypertension in PBC patients[1,2]. Hemodynamically, the site of the major resistance is mainly located at the presinusoidal level, particularly in the early stages of the disease. Thus, a gradient can exist between the portal vein pressure and the wedged hepatic vein pressure and, under such conditions, the hepatic vein pressure gradient may be much lower than the porto–hepatic pressure gradient[3,4].

The prevalence of portal hypertension may vary according to the way it is evaluated and also with the nature of referral. In most cases, portal hypertension is confirmed or inferred by the presence or absence of esophageal varices. However, portal hypertension can be present in the absence of varices and is only accurately measured by the determination of a porto–hepatic gradient, due to prehepatic type.

In 1987, Navasa et al.[5] found that 20 of 32 PBC patients (62.5%) had esophageal varices and/or an hepatic vein pressure gradient higher than 6 mmHg. These patients were the first 32 patients with PBC referred for inclusion in a therapeutic clinical trial in Spain.

More recently, Lindor et al.[6] found that only 35 of 174 PBC patients (20.1%) had esophageal varices at inclusion in their large double-blind clinical trial on the effect of ursodeoxycholic acid (UDCA). The wide difference between these studies may be due not only to the method of measurement of portal hypertension in the Navasa study (which, in fact, underestimated the real porto–hepatic gradient) but also to the dates of the two studies: many more unsymptomatic patients with PBC are diagnosed nowadays than 10–15 years ago, particularly with the wide use of multianalysers.

Only one published study has addressed the progression of portal hypertension, once diagnosed: Gores et al.[7] reported in 1988 that, of 265 PBC patients included in the D-penicillamine trial, 83 developed new varices over a 7-year follow-up period, that is, 31% of the patients. There was a much higher and earlier occurrence of varices in patients with histologic stage IV disease: 16% by the end of the first year and 36% by the end of the third year. Of these 83 patients, 40 had episodes of variceal bleeding over the same period (48%). However bleeding occurred very soon after the development of varices: 33% by the end of the first year and 41% by the end of the third year.

In a recent preliminary report on their UDCA trial, Lindor et al.[6] found that, in the placebo group, new esophageal varices occurred in 12 of 48 patients (25%) without varices on inclusion and followed for 2 years and in 18 of the 24 patients (75%) followed for 4 years.

Thus, portal hypertension, as manifested by the development of esophageal varices, is a common finding in the follow-up of patients with PBC. New varices can develop in at least 25–30% of patients over a period of 4–6 years. The incidence of new varices seems higher in patients with marked fibrosis on biopsy, although no correlation has been clearly defined between the degree of portal hypertension and the histological stage.

In order to evaluate the real incidence of portal hypertension in a large cohort of PBC patients, and particularly the effect of UDCA treatment on the progression of portal hypertension, we measured the porto–hepatic gradient at the time of referral to our clinic and then prospectively every second year.

PATIENTS AND METHODS

The study was performed in one hundred and one patients with primary biliary cirrhosis (PBC) referred to our out-patient clinic for the diagnosis of their liver disease. Eighty-eight were females and 13 were males, with ages ranging from 36 to 74 years (mean $\pm$ SD: 54 $\pm$ 10 y). The diagnosis of PBC was based on clinical and biochemical features of chronic cholestasis, presence of antimitochondrial antibodies and by compatible histological changes on liver biopsies. Only patients referred for liver transplantation and for whom treatment with UDCA was not considered were excluded from our study.

All patients were then followed at the out-patient clinic at regular intervals.

Portal hypertension was measured at the time of initial liver biopsy, and thereafter every 2 years. Free portal vein pressure and free hepatic vein pressure were recorded using a Chiba needle by the transcostal approach, performed under fluoroscopy and confirmed by contrast injections[4]. The porto–hepatic gradient was calculated as the difference between portal vein pressure and hepatic vein pressure.

In all patients, the aminopyrine breath test[8], used as a dynamic evaluation of liver function, was measured by the cumulative output of radioactive CO_2 in breath during a 2-hour collection period, and was expressed as per cent of the oral loading dose. This test was performed on inclusion in the study, then every year thereafter.

RESULTS

Inclusion data

There was a wide range in biochemical parameters, as typically found in PBC patients; in particular: AST: 89 ± 66 IU/L ($n < 32$); ALT: 99 ± 94 IU/L ($n < 38$); alkaline phosphatase: 463 ± 263 IU/L ($n < 94$); γ-GT: 597 ± 496 IU/L ($n < 60$); bilirubin: 16 ± 10 μmol/L ($n < 17$).

The aminopyrine breath test varied from 3.8% to 23.6% in the 101 patients (mean; 10.6 ± 3.7%); a value higher than 6% is considered normal in our laboratory.

The porto–hepatic gradient varied widely in the 101 patients from 1 to 26 mmHg. It was higher than 6 mmHg, the upper limit of normal value, in 54 patients (53%), and was higher than 12 mmHg in 20 patients (20%), 12 mmHg being the dangerous limit for bleeding from esophageal varices.

There was no correlation between the porto–hepatic gradient and the biochemical parameters (AST, ALT, alkaline phosphatase, γ-GT and bilirubin), or with the aminopyrine breath test.

The histologic stage was stage I in two patients, stage II in 18, stage III in 18 and stage IV in 63 patients. The Mayo score varied between 1.7 and 7.9 (mean: 3.9 ± 1.0).

A significant correlation was found with the Mayo score ($r^2 = 0.29$, $p < 0.0001$), while a weak correlation was found with the histologic stage ($r^2 = 0.10$, $p < 0.005$), more probably due to variability in the blind biopsy (sampling error) than its histologic interpretation.

Finally, using a multiple regression analysis with age, duration of the disease, AST, alkaline phosphatase, bilirubin, histologic stage and the Mayo score as independent variables, only the Mayo score was selected as a significant independent predictor of the porto–hepatic gradient.

Long-term follow-up data

Of the 101 patients included in the long-term study, 47 had (or would have) completed 72 months' follow-up (6 years). Initially, 30 patients were included in the French double-blind clinical trial on UDCA: 15 were allocated to the UDCA group and 15 to the placebo group for the first 2 years of follow-up, and then all were treated with UDCA for an additional 4 years. The 17 other patients were treated with UDCA for 6 years after the initial evaluation.

Of the 47 patients who had or would have completed the 72 months' follow-up, 27 were indeed evaluated every 2 years for the full period. The 20 other patients could not be evaluated thoroughly: 2 patients were transplanted early after being put on UDCA; 6 patients died before the end of the 6-year period (2 of bleeding varices, 2 of stroke, 1 of hepatoma and 1 of brain tumor).

In 12 patients, the porto–hepatic gradient could not be measured on follow-up (5 patients refused, 2 patients had cancer, 1 patient had refractory ascites, 1 patient was on anticoagulation therapy, and, in 3 patients, measurement was not successful). However, the initial porto–hepatic gradient was similar in both groups of patients.

Of 27 patients followed every second year for 72 months, 9 were on placebo for the first 24 months, then on UDCA from 24 to 72 months and 18 were on UDCA from the initial evaluation. As previously reported by the clinical trials on UDCA, there was a rapid significant improvement in alkaline phosphatase and AST after UDCA, improvement which was delayed in the group initially on placebo. However, in both groups, there was no significant change in bilirubin levels nor in the aminopyrine breath test over the 72 months.

When considering the porto–hepatic gradient measured in 9 patients initially on placebo, this value increased significantly at 24 months from 7.4 to 9.8 mmHg ($p < 0.05$), then stabilized until 48 months and finally returned to inclusion values by the end of the 72 months. These values were not different from values obtained on inclusion 6 years earlier. By contrast, in the 18 patients on UDCA from the beginning, the porto–hepatic gradient remained stable over the 72 months of follow-up (6.7 to 6.6 mmHg (NS)). Comparisons between values were performed using repeated measure analysis of variance.

These findings are in accordance with those presented recently by Lindor et al.[6] in which they reported a lower incidence of new esophageal varices in patients included in the UDCA group than in patients included in the placebo group of their clinical trial.

SUMMARY

Portal hypertension is not an uncommon finding in patients referred for the initial diagnosis of primary biliary cirrhosis, but is rarely severe. In patients not treated with UDCA, a progressive and slowly developing portal hypertension appears to occur with time. In patients treated with UDCA, progression of portal hypertension can be slowed during the first 2 years of treatment and, eventually, can be reversed after prolonged treatment.

In addition to the biochemical improvement, delay in death and liver transplantation, UDCA treatment may decrease the ocurrence of portal hypertension and subsequently the risk of developing varices in PBC patients. However, unlike the rapid improvement observed in biochemical tests, such as markers of cholestasis and cytolysis, the onset of these beneficial effects after prolonged UDCA treatment is delayed.

References

1. Kew MC, Varma RR, Dos Santos HA, et al. Portal hypertension in primary biliary cirrhosis. Gut 1971;121:830–4.
2. Lebrec D, Sicot C, Degott C, et al. Portal hypertension and primary biliary cirrhosis. Digestion 1976;14:220–6.
3. Boyer T, Triger D, Horisawa M, et al. Direct transhepatic measurement of portal vein pressure using a thin needle. Comparison with wedged hepatic vein pressure. Gastroenterology 1977;72:584–9.

4. Pomier-Layrargues G, Kusielewicz D, Willems B, *et al.* Presinusoidal portal hypertension in non-alcoholic cirrhosis. Hepatology 1985;5:415–18.
5. Navasa M, Parés A, Bruguera M, *et al.* Portal hypertension in primary biliary cirrhosis. Relationship with histological features. J Hepatol 1987;5:292–8.
6. Lindor KD, Jorgensen RA, Dickson ER. Ursodeoxycholic acid delays the onset of esophageal varices in primary biliary cirrhosis. Hepatology 1996;22:125A.
7. Gores GJ, Wiesner RH, Dickson ER, *et al.* Prospective evaluation of esophageal varices in primary biliary cirrhosis: Development, natural history, and influence on survival. Gastroenterology 1988;96:1552–9.
8. Villeneuve JP, Infante-Rivard C, Ampelas M, *et al.* Prognostic value of the aminopyrine breath test in cirrhotic patients. Hepatology 1986;6:928–31.

11
Management of primary biliary cirrhosis: osteoporosis

A. PARÉS

INTRODUCTION

Primary biliary cirrhosis (PBC) is a chronic cholestasic liver disease of unknown etiology, although the association with a large number of auto-immune disorders suggests that the disease may be of autoimmune origin. The disease usually affects middle-aged women and progresses from asymp-tomatic disease with only laboratory abnormalities to a severe cholestasic disease with deep jaundice, xanthomas, portal hypertension and eventually liver failure[1].

Bone disease complicates the natural history in patients with PBC. Indeed, osteopenia has noteworthy deleterious consequences, particularly because the final treatment for the disease is liver transplantation which may impair bone mass[2,3], and therefore, patients are prone to develop fractures. These consequences may be still more evident in patients treated with corticoste-roids for preventing liver rejection.

Osteodystrophy in patients with PBC was recognized soon after the first descriptions of the disease[4-13]. Initially, and probably because PBC patients were diagnosed at late stages of the disease with severe cholestasis, osteoma-lacia[5,6], which presumably resulted from low plasma vitamin D levels as a consequence of intestinal malabsorption, was common. Later on, patients were diagnosed at early stages, that is with mild cholestasis, and, therefore, osteomalacia is found very rarely in PBC[14-19].

INCIDENCE OF BONE DISEASE IN PBC

The incidence of bone disease in PBC has varied since the first description because of two main factors: the criteria used for diagnosing osteoporosis and osteomalacia and also because patients are now diagnosed at early stages of the disease and most of them are asymptomatic. In the initial studies the incidence of bone disease was assessed by X-rays of the spine, or by bone biopsy and histomorphometry[6,9-17]. However, in the last decade

Table 1 Prevalence of metabolic bone disease in primary biliary cirrhosis

Author, year, reference	Diagnostic procedures	Number of cases	Osteoporosis (%)	Osteomalacia (%)
Kehayoglou, 1968 [5]	Biopsy, X-rays	12	83	8
Compston, 1977 [6]	Biopsy	11	na	36
Brancós, 1979 [7]	X-rays	14	57	na
Compston, 1980 [8]	Biopsy, X-rays	30	40	10
Herlong, 1982 [12]	Biopsy, densitometry	15	67	0
Matloff, 1982 [10]	Biopsy, densitometry	10	60	0
Cuthbert, 1984 [11]	Biopsy	11	9	0
Hodgson, 1985 [13]	Densitometry	13	38	0
Stellon, 1987 [14]	Biopsy	12	37	0
Mitchison, 1988 [15]	Densitometry, biopsy	25	12	4
Guañabens, 1990 [17]	Biopsy	20	35	0
Lindor, 1995 [18]	Densitometry	180	35	na
Guañabens, 1997 [19]	Densitometry	100	27	na

na: not applicable.

bone mass has been best assessed by bone densitometry, mainly using dual energy X-ray absorptiometry[18,19] of the lumbar spine, proximal femur, and forearm. These techniques are more sensitive, reliable and accurate than bone histomorphometry for assessing osteoporosis, although bone biopsy with double tetracycline labeling is mandatory for establishing the diagnosis of osteomalacia, as well as to determine the rate of bone turnover.

Osteomalacia is now very uncommon in PBC, although originally most patients with symptoms of bone disease were considered to have osteomalacia after performing bone biopsy. The criteria for osteomalacia were not very well defined, although most patients had low plasma vitamin D levels which may account for this bone disease in patients with PBC[5,6]. Actually, in series from the seventies, the prevalence of osteomalacia was as high as 36% of cases[6], whereas ten years later, osteomalacia was only observed in one of 25 patients[15]. In our experience, true osteomalacia was not found in any patient with PBC[17] (Table 1).

Osteoporosis has emerged as the main metabolic bone disease in patients with PBC. Using the histomorphometric procedure, the prevalence of osteoporosis ranges from 9 to 60% of cases (Table 1). However, in the most relevant studies, the prevalence of osteoporosis is around 35% of cases[13,14,17]. These later prevalences of osteoporosis diagnosed through bone histomorphometry are very similar to those observed using densitometric procedures[18,19] (Table 1). In fact, the prevalence of osteoporosis in a series of 100 patients with PBC, using the criteria of lumbar or femoral bone mineral density lower than −2.5 T-scores (standard deviation below the adult mean value), was 27%[19], a figure very similar to that observed in another large series of patients with PBC from the United States[18].

One study, which focused on assessing the factors which influence the development of metabolic bone disease, found that osteoporosis in PBC was associated with duration of the liver disease, calcium malabsorption, and postmenopausal condition[17]. In contrast, osteoporosis was not related to the degree of cholestasis, measured by standard liver tests, such as bilirubin, alkaline phosphatase, and bile salt concentrations, although bilirubin levels were higher in patients with osteoporosis. Accordingly, it was postulated that the duration of cholestasis is more important than its severity for developing osteoporosis. Since most patients with PBC who had osteoporosis were postmenopausal, it could be questioned whether the development of bone loss was related to estrogen deficiency, more than PBC itself. However, the prevalence of osteoporosis is significantly higher in patients with PBC than in age-matched healthy controls who are also postmenopausal[19], thus indicating that liver disease plays a relevant role leading to increased bone loss. Osteoporosis is also related to intestinal calcium malabsorption, particularly in patients with lower circulating 25-hydroxyvitamin D levels, thus proving the consequences of chronic cholestasis in the development of osteoporosis.

Agents used for treatment of liver disease may also affect bone mass. As demonstrated in a controlled trial, treatment with prednisolone for one year adversely affected bone, since femoral absorptiometry fell 3.5%, as did trabecular bone volume assessed by histomorphometry[15]. Cyclosporin also influences bone turnover in patients with PBC, thus increasing bone formation and bone resorption, but delaying bone loss. Indeed, lumbar bone mineral density (BMD) did not change in patients taking cyclosporin, whereas it decreased markedly in patients with placebo[20,21]. Ursodeoxycholic acid (UDCA) is effective for preventing progression of PBC and retards the need for liver transplantation[22-26]. Preliminary data also indicate that treatment with UDCA tends to reduce the rate of bone loss in patients with PBC, although, after three years of treatment, UDCA was not associated with statistically significant differences in the rate of bone loss in the lumbar spine when compared with placebo despite the beneficial effects of UDCA on underlying liver disease[18].

BONE TURNOVER IN PBC

The actual amount of bone depends on the balance between two opposite mechanisms: bone formation induced by the osteoblasts and bone resorption caused by the osteoclasts. In patients with PBC, the mechanisms resulting in osteoporosis are not completely elucidated since some studies indicate an increased bone resorption (high-turnover osteoporosis) whereas other studies have suggested decreased bone formation (low-turnover osteoporosis). Actually, some bone histomorphometric studies have revealed increased bone resorption and turnover even in the absence of osteoporosis as an early feature of bone disease in PBC[12]. However, there are plenty of data showing impaired osteoblastic function resulting in lower mean wall thickness and defects in matrix synthesis, as well as a low bone formation rate[14,17]. This was observed in one histomorphometric analysis of transiliac bone biopsies in a series of 20 patients with PBC[17]. The bone formation rate was depressed in all but four patients (Figure 1). These morphometric data are consistent with decreased circulating levels of osteocalcin[20,21], a non-

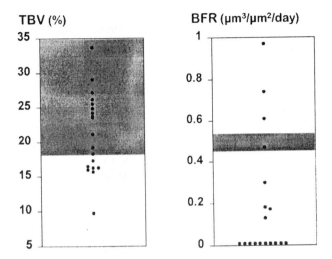

Figure 1 Trabecular bone volume (TBV) and bone formation rate (BFR) in a series of 20 patients with PBC[17]. Shaded areas indicate normal values.

collagenous bone protein considered a useful biochemical marker of bone turnover[27].

Although no conclusive data are available for explaining such discrepancies, patent or subtle calcium and vitamin D deficiencies leading to secondary hyperparathyroidism have been proposed as the causes of increased bone turnover found in some patients with PBC[13]. The low bone turnover in patients with normal calcium and vitamin D levels is secondary to impaired osteoblast function, perhaps related to the presence of factors normally metabolized or excreted by the liver but retained in cholestasis. In this respect, recent experimental data support the hypothesis that hyperbilirubinemia or possibly other substances impair osteoblast proliferative capacity and thus may play a major role in the pathogenesis of osteoporosis in patients with chronic cholestatic liver disease[28].

MANAGEMENT OF OSTEOPOROSIS IN PBC

Calcium and vitamin D

Vitamin D deficiency is nowadays very uncommon in patients with PBC, at least in countries such as Spain and in most areas of the United States with high rates of sunlight irradiation. However, since low 25-hydroxyvitamin D levels can be found in those patients with the most severe liver disease, oral supplements of this vitamin are appropriate for preventing osteomalacia. When patients are usually treated with 20–40 μg/day of 25-hydroxyvitamin D orally, all of them remain with normal circulating vitamin D levels, without evidence of intoxication.

Since intestinal calcium malabsorption is frequent in PBC, calcium supplements should be recommended to all patients. Depending on the daily intake of dairy products, which are the main source of dietary calcium, patients should receive between 1 and 1.5 g of oral elemental calcium per day. Oral calcium carbonate or gluconate is easily administered and well tolerated. Other sources of calcium, such as hydroxyapatite, have been considered more beneficial[29], although this has not been confirmed. Intravenous infusions of calcium gluconate have also been used for relieving bone pain secondary to osteopenia.

Despite adequate amounts of calcium and vitamin D supplements, patients with PBC continue to lose bone mass at a rate between 1 and 3% per year, depending on the menopausal state as well as baseline bone mineral density[19].

Sodium fluoride

Sodium fluoride stimulates bone formation and increases cancellous bone mass in postmenopausal osteoporosis[30-33], although discrepancies concerning the safety and antifracture efficacy of this agent have emerged. Since low bone formation rate is the main cause of osteoporosis in PBC, we examined the effects of sodium fluoride on bone mass in 22 patients with PBC in a placebo-controlled trial[34]. Eleven patients were randomly allocated into each group, either receiving 50 mg of sodium fluoride daily, or placebo for two years. Seven patients in the fluoride group and 8 patients in the placebo group completed the trial. Bone mass decreased markedly in the placebo group (initial: 1.00 ± 0.07, final: 0.93 ± 0.06 g/cm^2; $p = 0.03$), an effect which was observed after only 12 months. By contrast, in the fluoride group, bone mineral density did not change during the two-year period (initial: 1.05 ± 0.07, final: 1.07 ± 0.06 g/cm^2; NS). Moreover, lumbar BMD in the fluoride group increased by $3.1 \pm 3.5\%$ and, in the placebo group, decreased by $6.6 \pm 2.7\%$ ($p = 0.04$) (Figure 2). No patient in either group developed new vertebral or non-vertebral fractures. Side-effects were observed in 3 patients in the fluoride group, consisting mainly of epigastric pain and nausea. These results indicate that sodium fluoride prevents bone loss in patients with PBC.

Cyclical etidronate

Intermittent cyclical etidronate, an organic bisphosphonate compound which inhibits osteoclast-mediated bone resorption, has proven to be useful for the treatment of osteopenia. This drug increases spinal bone mass and reduces the incidence of further vertebral fractures in women with postmenopausal osteoporosis, without significant adverse effects[35,36]. Therefore, the effects of intermittent cyclical etidronate versus sodium fluoride on bone density and mineral metabolism in women with primary biliary cirrhosis have been compared in a clinical trial[37].

Patients received 400 mg/day of oral etidronate for two weeks, followed by a 13-week period without etidronate, or 50 mg of oral sodium fluoride (given as 25-mg enteric-coated tablets twice a day). All patients received calcium supplements and low doses of oral vitamin D. Sixteen patients were randomly allocated to each group which were similar with respect to clinical, biochemical and densitometric data. Thirteen patients in the etidronate

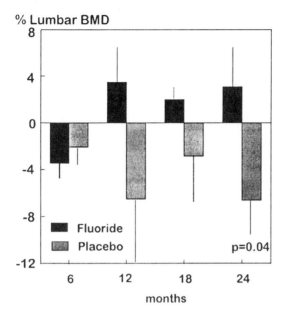

Figure 2 Changes in the lumbar bone mineral density induced by treatment with fluoride or placebo for 24 months.

group and 10 in the fluoride group completed the 2-year trial. In the etidronate group lumbar BMD increased significantly and femoral BMD did not change over two years. In the fluoride group, lumbar BMD did not change significantly after two years, but femoral BMD decreased, particularly in the Ward's triangle (Figures 3 and 4). Lumbar BMD in the etidronate group increased by $0.53 \pm 1.06\%$ while, in the fluoride group, it decreased by $1.94 \pm 2.54\%$. Conversely, bone density in the greater trochanter and Ward's triangle decreased in patients taking fluoride $(-5.84 \pm 2.3\%)$, whilst no changes were observed in patients taking etidronate $(-0.4 \pm 1.9\%)$. No patient on etidronate but two patients on fluoride developed new vertebral fractures. The number of patients developing further non-vertebral fractures was similar in both groups (3 patients receiving etidronate and 2 patients with fluoride). No significant adverse effects were observed in patients taking etidronate or fluoride, except for gastric symptoms in three patients treated with fluoride who left the trial.

This trial demonstrates that cyclical etidronate is more effective than sodium fluoride for preventing bone loss in patients with PBC receiving appropriate supplementation with calcium and vitamin D. The effects of etidronate were, indeed, better than those of fluoride, since spinal bone mineral density increased in patients receiving etidronate but decreased in patients with fluoride. This impairment was, however, lower than the 6.6% expected two-year bone loss in PBC patients taking only calcium and vitamin D supplements[34]. Moreover, etidronate prevented bone loss in the proximal femur, an effect which was not observed with fluoride. These effects

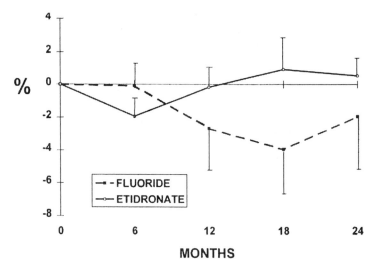

Figure 3 Changes in the lumbar bone mineral density induced by fluoride or etidronate for 24 months[34].

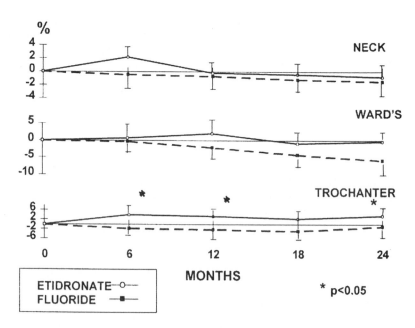

Figure 4 Changes in the femoral bone mineral density induced by fluoride or etidronate for 24 months[37]. * indicates $p < 0.05$ vs. baseline levels.

on bone mass paralleled the decreased bone remodeling as shown by a significant decline in urinary hydroxyproline and serum osteocalcin levels after two years of treatment with etidronate.

The best effects induced by etidronate on bone mass do not necessarily indicate that osteoporosis in PBC is of high bone turnover. It could merely reflect an effect on decreasing bone resorption which overcomes the depressed bone formation observed in patients with PBC. Despite the fact that this series includes only a small number of patients, we believe etidronate can now be the agent of choice for preventing bone loss in patients with PBC, in addition to calcium and vitamin D supplementation. Actually, cyclical etidronate also prevents bone loss associated with prednisone treatment in patients with PBC[38].

Calcitonin

Calcitonin inhibits osteoclastic bone resorption and has been used for preventing osteoporosis in a wide range of clinical conditions, particularly postmenopausal osteoporosis. The effect of this agent has also been studied in patients with PBC. In the first pilot study treatment with calcitonin, vitamin D and calcium in eleven patients resulted in a lower decrease in bone mineral density ($-0.91 \pm 7\%$) than in the 13 untreated patients, who experienced a marked derangement in their bone mass ($-4.93 \pm 8\%$) after 12 months[39]. The same group has recently published the long-term effects of this treatment which apparently was effective in patients with severe osteopenia[40]. These results were not confirmed in another well-conducted study which indicated that parenterally administered calcitonin for six months was ineffective in halting trabecular bone loss[41]. However, it should be taken into account that the patients were very osteopenic with a mean T-score below -2.5 and that the period of treatment was very short.

Since the effects of calcitonin, if any, for preventing bone loss in patients with PBC are less prominent than those observed with sodium fluoride or cyclical etidronate, the further potential of calcitonin is quite limited.

Estrogens

Estrogen replacement therapy is an effective treatment for preventing bone loss in postmenopausal women. No controlled trial has been performed in patients with PBC, but potential favorable effects of estrogens on bone mass of PBC patients have been reported[42]. Changes in lumbar spine bone mineral density were indeed significantly higher in a group of 16 postmenopausal patients treated with estrogens than in 91 postmenopausal PBC patients who did not receive estrogen replacement. Treatment with estrogens did not have any effect on clinical and biochemical cholestasis in these patients, thus suggesting that estrogen replacement may be an alternative procedure for preventing bone loss in patients with PBC and other chronic cholestatic diseases. However, since this information was retrospective, controlled trials are mandatory.

SUMMARY AND CONCLUSIONS

Osteoporosis is the main metabolic bone disease associated with PBC; osteomalacia is very uncommon. Although bone turnover may change during the disease, it is generally accepted that osteoporosis in PBC results from impaired osteoblast function probably as the consequence of cholestasis, and is particularly related to the duration of the disease, postmenopausal condition and intestinal calcium malabsorption. The management of osteoporosis is addressed to prevent the development of bone loss. Calcium and vitamin D supplements are mandatory, particularly in patients with severe cholestasis and in countries with a low rate of sunlight irradiation. Calcitonin has minor effects, if any, for preventing bone loss, whereas both sodium fluoride and cyclical etidronate are effective for treating trabecular osteopenia. Etidronate is more effective than sodium fluoride since it also prevents bone loss in the proximal femur, an effect which is not seen with fluoride. Despite these promising results, further studies including a larger number of patients treated with etidronate for longer periods, or using newer bisphosphonates with higher antiresorptive potency and less adverse effects on mineralization, or the combination of etidronate with estrogen replacement therapy are needed to substantially benefit patients with PBC.

References

1. Kaplan MM. Medical progress: primary biliary cirrhosis. N Engl J Med 1987;316:521-8.
2. Eastell R, Dickson ER, Hodgson SF, et al. Rates of vertebral bone loss before and after liver transplantation in women with primary biliary cirrhosis. Hepatology 1991;14:296-300.
3. Monegal A, Navasa M, Guanabens N, et al. Osteoporosis and bone mineral metabolism disorders in cirrhotic patients referred for orthotopic liver transplantation. Calcif Tissue Int 1997;60:148-54
4. Atkinson M, Nordin BEC, Sherlock S. Malabsorption and bone disease in prolonged obstructive jaundice. Q J Med 1956;99:299-312.
5. Kehayoglou AK, Holdsworth CD, Agnew JE, Whelton MJ, Sherlock S. Bone disease and calcium absorption in primary biliary cirrhosis. Lancet 1968;1:715-19.
6. Compston JE, Thompson RPH. Intestinal absorption of 25-hydroxyvitamin D and osteomalacia in primary biliary cirrhosis. Lancet 1977;1:721-4.
7. Brancós MA, Parés A, Bartrons S, et al. Las manifestaciones osteoarticulares en la cirrosis biliar primaria. Rev Esp Reumatol 1979;6:82-9.
8. Compston JE, Crowe JP, Wells IP, et al. Vitamin D prophylaxis and osteomalacia in chronic cholestatic liver disease. Dig Dis Sci 1980;25:28-32.
9. Arnaud SB. 25-Hydroxyvitamin D3 treatment of bone disease in primary biliary cirrhosis. Gastroenterology 1982;83:137-40.
10. Matloff DS, Kaplan MM, Neer RM, Goldberg MJ, Bitman W, Wolfe HJ. Osteoporosis in primary biliary cirrhosis: effects of 25-hydroxyvitamin D3 treatment. Gastroenterology 1982;83:97-102.
11. Cuthbert JA, Pak CYC, Zerwekh JE, Glass KD, Combes B. Bone disease in primary biliary cirrhosis: increased bone resorption and turnover in the absence of osteoporosis or osteomalacia. Hepatology 1984;4:1-8.
12. Herlong HF, Recker RR, Maddrey WC. Bone disease in primary biliary cirrhosis: histologic features and response to 25-hydroxyvitamin D. Gastroenterology 1982;83:103-8.
13. Hodgson SF, Dickson ER, Wahner HW, Johnson KA, Mann KG, Riggs BL. Bone loss and reduced osteoblast function in primary biliary cirrhosis. Ann Intern Med 1985;103:855-60.
14. Stellon AJ, Webb A, Compston J, Williams R. Low bone turnover state in primary biliary cirrhosis. Hepatology 1987;7:137-42.
15. Mitchison HC, Malcolm AJ, Bassendine MF, James OFW. Metabolic bone disease in primary biliary cirrhosis at presentation. Gastroenterology 1988;94:463-70.
16. Diamond TH. Metabolic bone disease in primary biliary cirrhosis. J Gastroenterol Hepatol 1990;5:66-81.
17. Guañabens N, Parés A, Mariñoso L, et al. Factors influencing the development of metabolic bone disease in primary biliary cirrhosis. Am J Gastroenterol 1990;85:1356-62.

18. Lindor KD, Janes CH, Crippin JS, Jorgensen Ram Dickson ER. Bone disease in primary biliary cirrhosis: Does ursodeoxycholic acid make a difference? Hepatology 1995;21:389–92.

19. Guañabens N, Parés A, Rodés J. Bone mineral density in primary biliary cirrhosis (unpublished data).

20. Guañabens N, Parés A, Navasa M, Ribera F, Muñoz J, Rodés J. Influencia de la ciclosporina A en el metabolismo óseo de la cirrosis biliar primaria. Rev Esp Reumatol 1990;17:14–5(abstract).

21. Guañabens N, Parés A, Navasa M, et al. Cyclosporin A increases the biochemical markers of bone remodeling in primary biliary cirrhosis. J Hepatol 1994;21:24–8.

22. Poupon Poupon RE, Balkau B, et al. A multicenter, controlled trial of ursodiol for the treatment of primary biliary cirrhosis. N Engl J Med 1991;324:1548–54.

23. Heathcote EJ, Cauch-Dudek K, Walker V, et al. The Canadian multicenter double-blind randomized controlled trial of ursodeoxycholic acid in primary biliary cirrhosis. Hepatology 1994;19:1149–56.

24. Lindor KD, Dickson ER, Baldus WP, et al. Ursodeoxycholic acid in the treatment of primary biliary cirrhosis. Gastroenterology 1994;106:1284–90.

25. Poupon RE, Poupon R, Balkau B and the UDCA-PBC Study Group. Ursodiol for the longterm treatment of primary biliary cirrhosis. N Engl J Med 1994;330:1342–7.

26. Parés A. Long-term treatment of primary biliary cirrhosis with ursodeoxycholic acid: Results of a randomized, double-blind, placebo-controlled trial. J Hepatol 1997;26; S166(abstract).

27. Price PA, Parthermore JG, Deftos LJ. New biochemical marker for bone metabolism. J Clin Invest 1980; 66:878–83.

28. Janes CH, Dickson ER, Okazaki R, Bonde S, McDonagh AF, Riggs BL. Role of hyperbilirubinemia in the impairment of osteoblast proliferation associated with cholestatic jaundice. J Clin Invest 1995;95:2581–6.

29. Epstein O, Kato Y, Dick R, Sherlock S. Vitamin D, hydroxyapatite, and calcium gluconate in treatment of cortical bone thinning in postmenopausal women with primary biliary cirrhosis. Am J Clin Nutr 1982;36:426–30.

30. Mamelle N, Meunier JP, Dusan R, et al. Risk–benefit of sodium fluoride treatment in primary vertebral osteoporosis. Lancet 1988;2:361–5.

31. Heaney RP, Baylink DJ, Johnston C, et al. Fluoride therapy for the vertebral crush fracture syndrome. A status report. Ann Intern Med 1989;111:678–80.

32. Riggs BL, Hodgson SF, O'Fallon WM, et al. Effect of fluoride treatment on the fracture rate in postmenopausal women with osteoporosis. N Engl J Med 1990;322:802–9.

33. Pak CYC, Sakhaee K, Adams-Huet B, Piziak V, Peterson RD, Poindexter JR. Treatment of postmenopausal osteoporosis with slow-release sodium fluoride. Final report of a randomized controlled trial. Ann Intern Med 1995;123:401–8.

34. Guañabens N, Parés A, Del Río L, et al. Sodium fluoride prevents bone loss in primary biliary cirrhosis. J Hepatol 1992;15:345–9.

35. Storm T, Thamsborg G, Steiniche T, Genant HK, Sorensen OH. Effect of intermittent cyclical etidronate therapy on bone mass and fracture rate in women with postmenopausal osteoporosis. N Engl J Med 1990;322:1265–71.

36. Watts NB, Harris ST, Genant HK, et al. Intermittent cyclical etidronate treatment of postmenopausal osteoporosis. N Engl J Med 1990;323:73–9.

37. Guañabens N, Parés A, Monegal A, et al. Etidronate versus fluoride for treatment of osteopenia in primary biliary cirrhosis: preliminary results after 2 years. Gastroenterology 1997;113:219–24.

38. Wolfhagen FH, Van Buuren HR, Den Ouden JW, et al. Cyclical etidronate in the prevention of bone loss in corticosteroid-treated primary biliary cirrhosis. A prospective, controlled trial. J Hepatol 1997;26:325–30.

39. Floreani A, Chiaramonte M, Giannini S, et al. Longitudinal study on osteodystrophy in primary biliary cirrhosis (PBC) and a pilot study on calcitonin treatment. J Hepatol 1991;12:217–23.

40. Floreani A, Zappala F, Fries W, et al. A 3-year pilot study with 1,25-dihydroxyvitamin D, calcium, and calcitonin for severe osteodystrophy in primary biliary cirrhosis. J Clin Gastroenterol 1997;24:239–44.

41. Camisasca M, Crosignani A, Battezzati PM, et al. Parenteral calcitonin for metabolic bone disease associated with primary biliary cirrhosis. Hepatology 1994;20:633–7.

42. Crippin JS, Jorgensen Ram Dickson ER, Lindor KD. Hepatic osteodystrophy in primary biliary cirrhosis: Effects of medical treatment. Am J Gastroenterol 1994;89:47–50.

12
Fatigue in the primary biliary cirrhosis patient

M. G. SWAIN

FATIGUE IN PRIMARY BILIARY CIRRHOSIS

Fatigue can be defined as "that state following a period of mental or bodily activity, characterized by a lessened capacity for work and reduced efficiency of accomplishment, usually accompanied by a feeling of weariness, sleepiness or irritability"[1].

The complaint of fatigue is common in patients with primary biliary cirrhosis (PBC) occurring in anywhere from 68% to 86% of patients[2-5]. Furthermore, fatigue in PBC has a significant impact upon the quality of life of these patients, constituting the worst symptom in almost one half of PBC patients[4] and ascribed to causing severely disabling effects on daily life in one quarter of PBC patients[4]. In fact, fatigue scores in 25–30% of PBC patients are similar to those which have been documented in patients with multiple sclerosis[4,5].

The complaint of fatigue in PBC patients does not appear to correlate with stage of disease, liver biochemistry, Mayo risk score, duration of, or response to ursodeoxycholic acid therapy[3-5]. However, fatigue in PBC patients does seem to be strongly associated with depression and obsessive–compulsive/somatization behavior[3-5], similar to that which has been observed in patients with chronic fatigue syndrome[6,7]. Interestingly, the obsessive–compulsive scores were the best predictors of fatigue score in PBC patients less than 45 years of age, and depression scores were the best predictors of fatigue scores in PBC patients over 45 years of age[4].

The etiology of fatigue in PBC patients is not understood, and, given the subjective nature of the complaint of fatigue, this area has received little scientific research attention. However, a recent study has demonstrated that the complaint of fatigue in PBC patients is central, not peripheral, in origin[8]. Specifically, Jalan et al. examined peripheral muscle fatigue in PBC patients by using electromyography and assessed central fatigue by using a battery of questionnaires[8]. No significant differences were noted in electromyography studies in PBC patients compared with normal volunteers; however, the

PBC patients demonstrated higher fatigue scores on the questionnaires and Jalan *et al.* interpreted these findings as being consistent with a defect in central neurotransmission as a probable underlying cause of fatigue in PBC patients[8]. This suggestion is supported by the findings of other groups which suggest a close link between central symptomatology (e.g. depression, somatization) and fatigue in PBC patients[3-5].

THEORETICAL CAUSES OF CENTRAL FATIGUE

The specific causes of central fatigue have not been well characterized. However, a number of theoretical causes of central fatigue have been suggested and investigated in patients with chronic fatigue syndrome and these theories are possibly applicable to patients with PBC. They can be defined within three major categories which will be discussed in detail: (a) neuroendocrine causes, (b) neurotransmitters and (c) immune activation/cytokines.

Neuroendocrine causes

Abnormalities in the function of the hypothalamic–pituitary–adrenal (HPA) axis have been observed in patients with chronic fatigue syndrome, fibromyalgia and seasonal affective disorder, all of which are characterized by fatigue[9-11]. These findings are suggestive of impaired central release of corticotropin-releasing hormone (CRH) in these conditions[9-11]. Neurons containing CRH project widely throughout the central nervous system in both man and animals. Furthermore, the central administration of CRH in rodents results in behavioral activation[12,13]. Therefore, a deficiency in the central release of CRH may contribute to the genesis of fatigue in PBC patients.

Neurotransmitters

Neuronal serotonin release within the central nervous system has been strongly implicated in the modification of mood and behavior. Furthermore, abnormalities in central serotonin release have been implicated in depression and obsessive–compulsive disorder, which are frequently observed in PBC patients and which correlate significantly with fatigue in these patients[3-5]. Serotonin is known to activate central CRH containing neurons and enhanced central sensitivity to serotonin has been documented in patients with chronic fatigue syndrome[14]. Moreover, some patients with chronic fatigue syndrome and fibromyalgia obtain improvement in their fatigue levels after treatment with medications which enhance central serotonergic neurotransmission[15]. Therefore, impaired central serotonin release or activity may contribute to fatigue in PBC patients.

Immune activation/cytokines

Proinflammatory cytokines (ie. IL-1, IL-6, TNFα), either released within the central nervous system or systemically, can modulate the activity of neural pathways within the brain which have been implicated in the genesis of fatigue (i.e. CRH and serotonin containing neurons[16,17]). In addition, elevated plasma cytokine levels have been observed in PBC patients and in cholestatic rats as well as in patients with chronic fatigue syndrome[18–20]. Furthermore, cytokines (especially IL-1β) have been implicated in the development of 'sickness behaviors' in rodents, including lethargy, fatigue and malaise[16]. Therefore, immune activation and cytokine release (either centrally or peripherally) in PBC patients may contribute to the symptoms of fatigue and lethargy seen in these patients.

EXPLORATION OF CENTRAL FATIGUE THEORIES IN AN ANIMAL MODEL OF CHOLESTASIS

Over the past 3–4 years, our laboratory has been systematically exploring these previously outlined theories of central fatigue genesis using a well-characterized rat model of cholestasis[21]. In this model, male Sprague–Dawley rats receive a laparotomy and then have their bile ducts manipulated only (sham controls) or ligated and resected (bile duct resected; BDR). This model reproducibly produces biochemical and clinical evidence of profound chole-stasis within 5 days[21], at which time the animals are studied.

Neuroendocrine (CRH)

BDR rats demonstrate decreased hypothalamic CRH levels, steady-state mRNA expression, and release compared with control animals[22]. Furthermore, BDR rats exhibit impaired stress-induced activation of their HPA axis compared with controls, again consistent with defective central CRH release in cholestatic animals[22]. Given these findings of impaired central CRH levels in BDR rats, we were interested in whether these observed abnormalities in CRH release contributed to the genesis of 'sickness beha-viors', like lethargy and fatigue, in these cholestatic animals. It has been previously observed that rats which have genetically determined impaired central CRH release behave in a specific manner when placed in an open field apparatus[23]. These congenitally CRH-deficient rats enter fewer squares in the center of the open field than normal rats[23]. We therefore used a similar open field apparatus (consisting of a flat area surrounded by 18-inch walls and divided into squares 7 inches wide) and sequentially placed BDR and sham control rats in it for a 5-min observation period[24]. BDR and sham rats entered a similar number of squares at the periphery of the field, indicating that the BDR animals did not have a global motor impairment. However, the BDR rats entered 50% fewer inner squares in the open field than did sham control rats[24], suggesting behavior consistent with defective central CRH release in the cholestatic animals. This suggestion was further supported by the observation that BDR animals dropped significantly fewer fecal pellets when exposed to the open field (considered a stressful stimulus) than did controls[24]. Central CRH release plays a critical role in stress-induced fecal boli production in rats[25] and these findings are consistent with defective central CRH release in cholestatic rats.

Therefore, defective central CRH release and associated defective CRH-mediated behaviors may contribute, at least in part, to cholestasis associated fatigue.

Neurotransmitters (serotonin)

Since central CRH release can be enhanced via serotonergic neurotransmission (through $5HT_{1A}$ receptors) and given that defective central serotonin neural activity has been implicated in the generation of fatigue, we next examined the potential beneficial effects of augmenting central $5HT_{1A}$ receptor activity upon fatigue in cholestatic rats. To do this, we adapted a swim test model of fatigue assessment[26]. The swim test measures the propensity of an animal to engage in, and capacity for, active behavior under conditions that are threatening and therefore highly motivating[26].

BDR and sham rats were treated with either vehicle or LY293284, a potent highly selective $5HT_{1A}$ receptor agonist, over a 24-h period, and then the rats were placed in the swim tank apparatus as described in detail previously[27]. Rats were observed over a 15-min period and the total times spent struggling, treading water, and floating motionless were recorded. From these recordings, an activity index (struggling time–floating time) was calculated for each rat. Vehicle-treated sham control rats struggled slightly more than they floated; however, vehicle-treated BDR rats floated strikingly more than they struggled[27]. Treatment of sham controls with LY293284 resulted in little change in their activity index. However, similar treatment of cholestatic rats resulted in a marked increase in their activity index, such that the activity index observed for vehicle-treated sham rats and LY293284-treated sham and BDR rats were no different[27].

Therefore, these data are consistent with the existence of defective $5HT_{1A}$-mediated neurotransmission in cholestatic rats which contributes to cholestasis-associated fatigue and can be corrected by enhancing $5HT_{1A}$ receptor activation in the central nervous system.

Immune activation (cytokines)

Cytokines can profoundly induce 'sickness behaviors', such as lethargy and fatigue, by acting at the level of the hypothalamus[16]. IL-1β released within the brain during illness has been most commonly implicated in the development of these symptoms[28,29]. Therefore, we speculated that, in cholestasis, changes may occur within the central nervous system which may result in enhanced sensitivity to these 'sickness behavior'-inducing properties of IL-1β. To examine this, we inserted intracerebroventricular (icv) cannulae into rats and 5 days later either bile duct resected or sham resected them. Five days after laparotomy, IL-1β (30 mg) or vehicle was infused icv and rats were placed in an open field 2 h later; the number of squares entered over a 5-min observation period was determined. Sham and BDR rats infused icv with vehicle entered the same number of squares during the observation period. Infusion of IL-1β icv resulted in a slight but insignificant drop in the number of squares entered by sham rats. However, IL-1β infusion in BDR rats resulted in a striking 70% drop in the number of squares entered during the observation period. These data suggest that cholestatic rats have enhanced central sensitivity to IL-1β-induced 'sickness behaviors'.

Therefore, enhanced central sensitivity to cytokines in cholestasis may contribute, at least in part, to the development of fatigue in PBC patients.

SUMMARY

In summary, cholestasis in the rat appears to be associated with a number of central defects which may potentially contribute to the development of fatigue. These defects include:

(a) Decreased central CRH release;
(b) Decreased central serotonergic neurotransmission; and
(c) Enhanced central sensitivity to IL-1β-induced 'sickness behaviors'.

The specific targeting of these defects may provide novel therapeutic interventions for treating fatigue in PBC patients.

References

1. Stedman's Medical Dictionary. Edn. 25. Baltimore: Williams and Wilkins; 1990.
2. Witt-Sullivan H, Heathcote J, Cauch K, et al. The demography of primary biliary cirrhosis in Ontario, Canada. Hepatology 1990;12:98–105.
3. Huet P-M, Deslauriers J, Faucher C, Charbonneau J. Fatigue, mental health and depression in patients with primary biliary cirrhosis (PBC). Hepatology 1996;24:A161.
4. Huet P-M, Deslauriers J. Impact of fatigue on quality of life of patients with primary biliary cirrhosis. Gastroenterology 1996;110:A1215.
5. Cauch-Dudek K, Abbey S, Stewart DE, Heathcote EJ. Fatigue and quality of life in primary biliary cirrhosis. Hepatology 1995;22:A6.
6. Wessely S, Powell R. Fatigue syndromes: A comparison of chronic 'postural' fatigue with neuromuscular and affective disorders. J Neurol Neurosurg Psychiatry 1989;42:940–8.
7. Blakely A, Howard R, Sosich R, Murdoch J, Menkes D, Spears G. Psychological symptoms, personality and ways of coping in chronic fatigue syndrome. Psychol Med 1991;21:347–62.
8. Jalan R, Gibson H, Lombard MG. Patients with PBC have central but no peripheral fatigue. Hepatology 1996;24:A162. ·
9. Demitrack MA, Dale JK, Straus SE, et al. Evidence for impaired activation of the hypothalamic–pituitary–adrenal axis in patients with chronic fatigue syndrome. J Clin Endocrinol Metab 1991;73:1224–34.
10. Griep E, Boersman J, de Kloet E. Altered reactivity of the hypothalamic–pituitary–adrenal axis in the primary fibromyalgia syndrome. J Rheumatol 1993;20:469–74.
11. Joseph-Vanderpool JR, Rosenthal NE, Chrousos GP, et al. Abnormal pituitary–adrenal responses to corticotropin-releasing hormone in patients with seasonal affective disorder: Clinical and pathophysiological implications. J Clin Endocrinol Metab 1991;72:1382–7.
12. Sutton RE, Koob GF, Le Moal M, Rivier J, Vale W. Corticotropin releasing factor produces behavioural activation in rats. Nature 1982;297:331–3.
13. Koob GF, Bloom FE. Corticotropin-releasing factor and behaviour. Fed Proc 1985; 44:259–63.
14. Bakheit AMO, Behan PO, Dinan TG, Gray CE, O'Keane V. Possible upregulation of hypothalamic 5-hydroxytryptamine receptors in patients with postural fatigue syndrome. Br Med J 1992;304:1010–12.
15. Goldenberg D, Mayskiy M, Mossey C, Ruthazer R, Schmid C. A randomized double-blind crossover trial of fluoxetine and amitriptylline in the treatment of fibromyalgia. Arthritis Rheum 1996;39:1852–9.
16. Kent S, Bluthe R-M, Kelly K, Dantzer R. Sickness behaviour as a new target for drug development. Trends Pharmacol Sci 1992;3:24–8.
17. Tsagarakis S, Gilles G, Rees L, Besser M, Grossman A. Interleukin-1 directly stimulates the release of corticotropin releasing factor from rat hypothalamus. Neuroendocrinology 1989;49:98–101.
18. Tilg H, Wilmer A, Vogel W, et al. Serum levels of cytokines in chronic liver diseases. Gastorenterology 1991;103:264–74.
19. Buchwald D, Wener MH, Pearlman T, Kith P. Markers of inflammation and immune activation in chronic fatigue and chronic fatigue syndrome. J Rheum 1991;24:372–6.

20. Swain MG, Appleyard CB, Wallace JL, Maric M. TNF-α facilitates inflammation-induced glucocorticoid secretion in rats with biliary obstruction. J Hepatol 1997;26:361–8.
21. Cameron GP, Oakley CL. Ligation of the common bile duct. J Pathol Bacteriol 1932; 35:769–98.
22. Swain MG, Patchev V, Vergalla J, Chrousos GP, Jones EA. Suppression of hypothalamic–pituitary–adrenal axis responsiveness to stress in a rat model of acute cholestasis. J Clin Invest 1993;91:1903–8.
23. Sternberg EM, Glowa JR, Smith MA, et al. Corticotropin-releasing hormone related behavioural and neuroendocrine responses to stress in Lewis and Fischer rats. Brain Res 1992;570:54–60.
24. Swain MG, Maric M. Defective corticotropin-releasing hormone mediated neuroendocrine and behavioural responses in cholestatic rats: Implications for cholestatic liver disease-related sickness behaviours. Hepatology 1995;22:1560–4.
25. Bonaz B, Tache Y. Water avoidance stress-induced c-fos expression in the rat brain and stimulation of fecal output: role of corticotropin-releasing factor. Brain Res 1994;641:21–8.
26. Weiss JM, Simson PG, Hoffman LJ, Abrose MJ, Cooper S, Webster A. Infusion of adrenergic receptor agonists and antagonists into the locus coeruleus and ventricular system of the brain effects on swim-motivated and spontaneous motor activity. Neuropharmacology 1986;25:367–84.
27. Swain MG, Maric M. Improvement in cholestasis-associated fatigue with a serotonin receptor agonist using a novel rat model of fatigue assessment. Hepatology 1997;25:291–4.
28. Kent S, Bluthe R-M, Dantzer R, et al. Different receptor mechanisms mediate the pyrogenic and behavioural effects of interleukin 1. Proc Natl Acad Sci USA 1992;89:9117–20.
29. Rothwell NJ, Hopkins SJ. Cytokines and the nervous system II: Actions and mechanisms of action. TINS 1995;18:130–6.

13
The pruritus of cholestasis: behavioral studies shed light on its pathogenesis

N. V. BERGASA AND E. A. JONES

Pruritus is a symptom experienced by 80% of patients with primary biliary cirrhosis (PBC)[1] and 20–60% of jaundiced patients[2]. The presence of pruritus or the degree to which it is experienced does not correlate with routine serum biochemical indices of cholestasis. It can be mild to severe and it does not tend to be easily relieved by scratching.

Pruritus in cholestatic patients is a difficult symptom to manage and its negative impact on the quality of life can be so severe that it can be an indication for liver transplantation[3].

The etiology of the pruritus of cholestasis is unknown. It has been considered to result from abnormally high plasma concentrations of substances that are normally secreted into bile. The reported rapid disappearance of pruritus in patients when large duct biliary obstruction is relieved is consistent with this suggestion. In addition, when cholestatic patients develop hepatocellular failure, pruritus usually subsides, suggesting that pruritogenic substances or cofactors of pruritogenic substances may be synthesized by the cholestatic liver[4].

Bile acids accumulate in the plasma of patients with cholestasis, and their intracutaneous administration under artificial conditions has been reported to induce pruritus[5,6]. These observations have suggested that bile acids mediate the pruritus of cholestasis. However, plasma concentrations of bile acids do not correlate with the pruritus of cholestasis[4].

Research on the pruritus of cholestasis has concentrated on the measurement of substances that circulate in the plasma of patients with cholestasis. However, this approach has not identified a specific group of substances that mediate this form of pruritus. Thus, the pruritus of cholestasis has been managed empirically and not satisfactorily (Reference 7 and references therein).

A coventional treatment for the pruritus of cholestasis has been the non-absorbable resins, cholestyramine and colestipol, which bind anions in the small intestine and decreases their enterohepatic circulation. Many patients appear to respond to this treatment with a decrease in their pruritus[8]; the response may be prolonged or transient, and some patients do not respond to this treatment at all.

The majority of treatments used for the pruritus of cholestasis lack a clear rationale (Reference 7 and references therein). Phenobarbital[9] and antihistamines[10] have been used frequently, but their effect on the pruritus of cholestasis may be non-specific, due to sedation rather than a specific reversal of factors contributing to pruritus. The xerostomia associated with antihistamines can worsen that of patients with PBC and Sjogren's syndrome.

The antibiotic rifampicin was reported to decrease the pruritus of cholestasis[11–13], although not consistently[14], in studies that applied subjective endpoints. The mechanism by which rifampicin decreases the pruritus of cholestasis is unknown. If rifampicin is used for this indication, the risk of hepatotoxicity associated with rifampicin therapy needs to be considered.

METHODOLOGICAL CONSIDERATIONS IN THE STUDY OF THE PRURITUS OF CHOLESTASIS

One of the major problems with research in the pruritus of cholestasis is that, because pruritus is a perception, it is difficult to study objectively. Pruritus is defined as the need to scratch and, because it is a perception, it cannot be directly quantitated. However, most people scratch when they itch. Accordingly, by quantitating this behavioral consequence of pruritus, an objective quantitative efficacy endpoint can be incorporated into the design of trials of therapies for the pruritus of cholestasis. The first attempts to measure scratching activity, more than a decade ago, involved the application of limb movement meters which did not measure scratching activity alone[15–17]. More recently, a scratching activity monitoring system has been devised which measures scratching activity independent of limb movements[18].

THE ENDOGENOUS OPIOID SYSTEM AND PRURITUS OF CENTRAL ORIGIN

Opioid receptors and endogenous opioid peptides are found in the central nervous system (CNS) and in peripheral nerves[19,20]. In addition, opioid peptides can be detected in some peripheral tissues[21]. Clinical and experimental data have revealed that compounds with agonist properties that exert their effects by binding to opioid receptors are associated with pruritus of neurogenic origin. The evidence is as follows:

(a) The intrathecal administration of the alkaloid morphine and opiate agonist drugs to humans is associated with pruritus, which is reversed by opiate antagonist drugs[22,23];

(b) The intracisternal administration of morphine to cats is associated with violent facial scratching[24]; and

(c) Microinjections of the opiate agonist analog DAMGO into the medullary dorsal horn of monkeys is associated with facial scratching that is prevented by naloxone[25].

These findings suggest that the increased opioidergic tone in the brain that results from the administration of agonist ligands of opioid receptors can result in pruritus and support the mediation of pruritus via a pathway that includes activation of opioid receptors.

In support of the existence of the concept of central neurogenic pruritus is the pruritus that complicates certain disorders of the CNS, such as multiple sclerosis, strokes, and space-occupying lesions (e.g. brain abscesses, tumors)[26-28].

INCREASED OPIOIDERGIC TONE IN CHOLESTASIS AND ITS RELATIONSHIP TO PRURITUS

Two lines of evidence suggest that there is increased opioidergic neurotransmission in cholestasis: (a) the administration of opiate antagonist drugs to patients with chronic liver disease is associated with an opiate withdrawal-like reaction[29,30]; and (b) rats with cholestasis secondary to bile duct resection (BDR), exhibit a state of antinociception, or analgesia, that is stereoselectively reversed by naloxone[31]. Thus, by analogy with the pruritus that can result from the pharmacological increase in central opioidergic neurotransmission[22-25], an increase in central opioidergic tone may also contribute to the pruritus of cholestasis. This concept is supported by ameliorations of the pruritus of cholestasis by opiate antagonist drugs (see below).

OPIATE ANTAGONIST DRUGS IN THE TREATMENT OF THE PRURITUS OF CHOLESTASIS

The use of an opiate antagonist drug for the treatment of the pruritus of cholestasis was first reported by Bernstein and Swift as a single experience with a patient with PBC and intractable pruritus[32], who responded to the administration of naloxone, but not saline, with transient disappearance of pruritus. Several years later, Thornton and Losowsky reported the disappearance of pruritus in nine patients with PBC after the administration of the oral opiate antagonist nalmefene[29].

Beneficial effects of opiate antagonists on the perception of pruritus and on scratching activity have been demonstrated in patients with cholestatic liver diseases. In a single-blind placebo-controlled study of eight patients with PBC, naloxone infusions were associated with a mean decrease in scratching activity of 50%[33]. These results were confirmed in a double-blind placebo-controlled study of 29 patients with the pruritus of cholestasis, 16 of whom had PBC[34]. The preferred route of administration of naloxone is the parenteral route because it has low bioavailability when administered orally[23,33,34]. Because the management of this form of pruritus may be long term, a drug that is bioavailable after oral administration would facilate the treatment. Nalmefene is bioavailable when administered orally and it has a good safety profile[35]. The effect of nalmefene on the perception of pruritus and scratching activity was studied in an open-label study and in a controlled blinded study of patients with cholestasis. In both studies, nalmefene administration was associated with a significant amelioration of the perception of pruritus and of scratching activity.

Recently, in a placebo-controlled study, the oral administration of the opiate antagonist naltrexone was reported to be associated with a decrease in the perception of pruritus[36]. There are concerns regarding the hepatotoxicity of naltrexone[37]; accordingly, its administration to these patients requires vigilance.

The specific mechanism responsible for increased opioidergic tone in cholestasis is unknown. One possibility is that there is increased availability of opioid peptides at opioid receptors in the central nervous system, where the signals responsible for pruritus are processed. In support of this concept is a decrease in the density of opioid receptors in the brain of rats with cholestasis secondary to BDR[38]. One possible source of opioid peptides in cholestasis is the liver, an organ that is not considered to be a source of endogenous opioid peptides under physiological conditions in adults. Three lines of evidence suggest that the cholestatic liver produces endogenous opioids:

(a) In the rat model of cholestasis secondary to BDR, but not in control livers, the mRNA of the gene that codes for Met-enkephalin and Met-enkephalin-containing peptides was found[39];

(b) Met-enkephalin immunoreactivity was detected in the cholestatic rat livers, which suggests complete processing of the mRNA message[39]; and

(c) Met-enkephalin immunoreactivity was also detected in livers from patients with PBC but not in livers from disease controls[40].

Thus, the cholestatic liver may directly contribute to the increased opioidergic tone of cholestasis by synthesizing biologically active opioid receptor agonist ligands.

Evidence has been obtained that plasma of cholestatic patients with pruritus contains a substance that induces opioid-receptor-mediated scratching activity of central origin. When plasma extracts from cholestatic patients with pruritus were microinjected into the medullary dorsal horn of monkeys, facial scratching was induced, which was prevented by naloxone but not by saline[41].

Although there is now ample evidence that opioidergic tone is increased in cholestasis and that this phenomenon contributes to the pruritus of cholestasis, the opioids responsible for mediating increased opioidergic tone and pruritus in cholestasis have not been identified.

THE SEROTONIN NEUROTRANSMITTER SYSTEM AND PRURITUS OF CHOLESTASIS

Like the opioid system, the serotonin system is also involved in the mediation of nociception[42]. Thus, by analogy with the opioid system, the use of a serotonin antagonist may be an alternative treatment for the pruritus of cholestasis. Although there are no definitive data demonstrating that serotoninergic neurotransmission is increased in cholestasis, experimental data suggest that increased central opioidergic tone can result in increased serotonergic tone[42,43].

Ondansetron is a drug that acts as an antagonist of the type 3 serotonin receptor (5-HT3) which is found in the CNS and on peripheral nerves[44]. In a placebo-controlled study of ten patients with the pruritus of cholestasis, two of whom had PBC, the bolus intravenous administration of ondansetron was reported to be followed by subjective ameliorations of pruritus that lasted for several hours[45]. In another study, nineteen patients with cholestasis and pruritus (17 of whom had PBC) were included; nine patients were randomized to receive placebo and 10 to receive ondansetron. The first dose of the study drug (or placebo) was administered intravenously, followed by the administration of the oral form for five days. Scratching activity was measured during the first 24 h after the intravenous treatment and the perception of pruritus was evaluated throughout the five-day treatment period. The effect of ondansetron on scratching activity and on the perception of pruritus was reported to be similar in both groups[46]. Considering the difference in the design of these two studies, their different results, and the facilitating role of serotonin in the mediation of nociception, studies of longer duration are necessary to clarify a possible role of this neurotransmitter in the pruritus of cholestasis.

CONCLUDING PERSPECTIVES

It is now apparent that increased opioidergic tone contributes to the pathophysiology of cholestasis and specifically to the pruritus of cholestasis, which may be, at least in part, centrally mediated.

The incorporation of an objective quantitative efficacy endpoint into the design of trials of therapies for the pruritus of cholestasis will enable the roles of specific substances or classes of substances in the pathogenesis of the pruritus of cholestasis to be defined more clearly.

References

1. Ghent CN. Cholestatic pruritus. In: Bernhard JD, ed. Itch Mechanisms and Managements of Pruritus. New York: McGraw-Hill, Inc; 1994:229-42.
2. Gleeson D, Boyer J. Intrahepatic cholestasis. In: McIntyre N, Benhamou J-P, Bircher J, Rizzetto M, Rodés J, eds. Oxford Textbook of Clinical Hepatology. New York: Oxford University Press; 1991:1087-107.
3. Elias E, Burra P. Primary biliary cirrhosis: symptomatic treatment. J Gastroenterol Hepatol 1991;6:570-3.
4. Lloyd-Thomas HGL, Sherlock S. Testosterone therapy for the pruritus of obstructive jaundice. Br Med J 1952;2:1289-91.
5. Schoenfield L, Sjovall J, Perman E. Bile acids on the skin of patients with pruritic hepatobiliary disease. Nature 1967;213:93-4.
6. Varadi DP. Pruritus induced by crude bile and purified bile acids. Experimental production of pruritus in human skin. Arch Dermatol 1974;109:678-81.
7. Bergasa NV, Jones EA. Management of the pruritus of cholestasis: potential role of opiate antagonists. Am J Gastroenterol 1991;86:1404-12.
8. Datta DV, Sherlock S. Cholestyramine for long term relief of the pruritus complicating intrahepatic cholestasis. Gastroenterology 1966;50:323-32.

9. Bloomer JR, Boyer JL. Phenobarbital effects in cholestatic liver diseases. Ann Intern Med 1975;82:310–17.
10. Duncan JS, Kennedy HJ, Triger DR. Treatment of pruritus due to chronic obstructive liver disease. Br Med J (Clin Res Ed) 1984;289:22.
11. Ghent CN, Carruthers SG. Treatment of pruritus in primary biliary cirrhosis with rifampin. Results of a double-blind, crossover, randomized trial. Gastroenterology 1988;94:488–93.
12. Bachs L, Parés A, Elena M, Piera C, Rodés J. Effects of long-term rifampicin administration in primary biliary cirrhosis. Gastroenterology 1992;102:2077–80.
13. Bachs L, Parés A, Elena M, Piera C, Rodés J. Comparison of rifampicin with phenobarbitone for treatment of pruritus in biliary cirrhosis. Lancet 1989;1:574–6.
14. Woolf GM, Reynold TB. Failure of rifampicin to relieve pruritus in chronic liver disease. J Clin Gastroenterol 1990;12:174–7.
15. Savin J, Paterson W, Oswald I. Scratching during sleep. Lancet 1973;2:296–7.
16. Felix R, Shuster S. A new method for the measurement of itch and the response to treatment. Br J Dermatol 1975;93:303–12.
17. Savin J, Paterson W, Oswald I, et al. Further studies of scratching during sleep. Br J Dermatol 1975;93:297–302.
18. Talbot TL, Schmitt JM, Bergasa NV, Jones EA, Walker EC. Application of piezo film technology for the quantitative assessment of pruritus. Biomed Instrum Technol 1991;25:400–3.
19. Blanchard SG, Chang KT. Regulation of opioid receptors. In: Pasternak G, ed. The Opiate Receptor. Clifton, NJ: Humana Press; 1988:425–39.
20. Jessell TM, Kelly DD. Pain and analgesia. In: Kandel ER, Schwartz JH, Jessell TM, eds. Principles of Neural Science. Third edn. Norwalk, Ct: Appleton & Lange; 1991:385–399.
21. Székely JI, Ramabadran K. Localization and ontogeny of opioid peptides and receptors. In: Opioid Peptides. Boca Raton: CRC Press; 1990:133–61.
22. Reiz S, Westberg M. Side effects of epidural morphine. Lancet 1980;2:203–4.
23. Jaffe J, Martin W. Opioid analgesics and antagonists. In: Gilman A, Goodman L, Rall T, eds. The Pharmacologic Basis of Therapeutics. 7th edn. New York: Macmillan; 1985:491–531.
24. Koenigstein H. Experimental study of itch stimuli in animals. Arch Dermatol Syphilol 1948;57:828–49.
25. Thomas DA, Williams GM, Iwata K, Kenshalo DJ, Dubner R. Effects of central administration of opioids on facial scratching in monkeys. Brain Res 1992;585:315–17.
26. Osterman P. Paroxysmal itching in multiple sclerosis. Br J Dermatol 1976;95:555–8.
27. Massey E. Unilateral neurogenic pruritus following stroke. Stroke 1984;15:901–3.
28. Sullivan M, Drake M. Unilateral pruritus and Nocardia brain abscess. Neurology 1984;123:1527–30.
29. Thornton JR, Losowsky MS. Opioid peptides and primary biliary cirrhosis. Br Med J 1988;297:1501–4.
30. Bergasa NV, Schmitt JP, Talbot TL, et al. Open-label trial of oral nalmefene for the pruritus of cholestasis. Hepatology 1998 (In press).
31. Bergasa NV, Alling DW, Vergalla J, Jones EA. Cholestasis in the male rat is associated with naloxone-reversible antinociception. J Hepatol 1994;20:85–90.
32. Bernstein JE, Swift R. Relief of intractable pruritus with naloxone. Arch Dermatol 1979;115:1366–7.
33. Bergasa NV, Talbot TL, Alling DW, et al. A controlled trial of naloxone infusions for the pruritus of chronic cholestasis. Gastroenterology 1992;102:544–9.
34. Bergasa NV, Alling DW, Talbot TL, et al. Naloxone ameliorates the pruritus of cholestasis: results of a double-blind randomized placebo-controlled trial. Ann Intern Med 1995;123:161–7.
35. Dixon R, Gentile J, Hsu H-B, et al. Nalmefene: safety and kinetics after single and multiple oral doses of a new opioid antagonist. J Clin Pharmacol 1987;27:233–9.
36. Wolfhagen FHJ, Sternieri E, Hop WCJ, Vitale G, Bertolotti M, van Buuren HR. Oral naltrexone treatment for cholestatic pruritus: a double-blind, placebo-controlled study. Gastroenterology 1997;113:1264–9.
37. Naltrexone. In: Physicians Desk Reference. 51st edn. Montvale, New Jersey: Medical Economics Company; 1996:957–9.

38. Bergasa NV, Rothman RB, Vergalla J, Xu H, Swain MG, Jones EA. Central mu-opioid receptors are down-regulated in a rat model of cholestasis. J Hepatol 1992;15:220–4.
39. Bergasa NV, Sabol SL, Young SW, Kleiner DE, Jones EA. Cholestasis is associated with preproenkephalin mRNA expression in the adult rat liver. Am J Physiol 1995;268:346–54.
40. Bergasa NV, Ghali V. Met-enkephalin immunoreactivity is expressed in the livers from patients with primary biliary cirrhosis (PBC). Gastroenterology 1997;26:441A.
41. Bergasa N, Thomas D, Vergalla J, Turner M, Jones E. Serum extracts from cholestatic patients induce naloxone-reversible centrally-mediated facial scratching in monkeys. Life Sci 1992;53:1253–8.
42. Richardson B. Serotonin and nociception. Ann NY Acad Sci 1990;600:511–20.
43. Kiefel JM, Cooper ML, Bodnar RJ. Serotonin receptor subtype antagonists in the medial ventral medulla inhibit mesencephalic opiate analgesia. Brain Res 1992;597:331–8.
44. Leonard B. Sub-types of serotonin receptors: biochemical changes and pharmacological consequences. Intern Clin Psychopharmacol 1992;7:13–21.
45. Schwöer H, Hartmann H, Ramadori G. Relief of cholestatic pruritus by a novel class of drugs: 5-hydroxytryptamine type 3 (5-HT3) receptor antagonists: effectiveness of ondansetron. Pain 1995;61:33–7.
46. O'Donohue JW, Haigh C, Williams R. Ondansetron in the treatment of the pruritus of cholestasis: a randomised controlled trial. Gastroenterology 1997;112:A1349.

14
Old and new immunosuppressant drugs: mechanisms and potential value

J. M. VIERLING

INTRODUCTION

Primary biliary cirrhosis (PBC) is a chronic, progressive cholestatic liver disease that predominantly affects women. It is characterized by inflammatory destruction of interlobular and septal bile ducts, periportal hepatitis, septal fibrosis and ultimately biliary cirrhosis[1,2]. The fundamental histopathologic lesion of the intrahepatic bile ducts in PBC is non-suppurative destructive cholangitis (NSDC) which is characterized by T cell infiltration of the biliary epithelia, resulting in segmental apoptosis of biliary epithelial cells and destruction of the bile duct[1-3]. Portal inflammatory infiltrates are predominantly composed of CD4 and CD8 T cells, and the CD4 T cells express a T helper 1 phenotype[4]. The observation that NSDC of interlobular and septal bile ducts also occurs in alloimmune-mediated conditions of hepatic allograft rejection and chronic graft-versus-host disease provides circumstantial support for the hypothesis that NSDC in PBC is mediated by autoimmune mechanisms[1,2]. Indeed, PBC has been considered a model autoimmune disease.

In contrast to classic autoimmune diseases, several features of PBC suggest that it may not be an autoimmune disease (Table 1). For example, PBC is observed only in adults and not in children, while all other autoimmune diseases occur in childhood[1]. As with classic autoimmune diseases, PBC is characterized by circulating autoantibodies, specifically antimitochondrial antibodies (AMA). However, in contrast to classic autoantibodies that react with diverse epitopes, the principal target of AMA is a highly restricted conformational epitope of the lipoyl domain of pyruvate dehydrogenase complex dihydrolipoamide acetyltransferase (PDC-E2)[5]. Most autoimmune diseases have strong HLA associations; however, PBC is only weakly associated with HLA DR8, and some patient populations do not exhibit this association[6]. Finally, PBC responds poorly to immunosuppressive medication[1], whereas other autoimmune diseases respond well.

Table 1 Comparative features of primary biliary cirrhosis and classic autoimmune diseases

	Classic autoimmunity	Primary biliary cirrhosis
Female bias	Yes	Yes
Age	Children and adults	Adults only
Autoantibodies	Yes	Yes
Autoantibody epitopes	Diverse	Restricted
HLA associations	Strong	Weak and only in minority
Associated autoimmune diseases	Yes	Yes
Response to immunosuppression	Good	Poor

There are several possible explanations for the poor response of PBC to immunosuppressants. First, the long natural history of PBC, including a preclinical stage of NSDC and AMA positivity in the absence of symptoms or biochemical abnormalities and an asymptotic stage in which up to 43% have biopsy evidence of cirrhosis when diagnosed[1], often results in diagnosis and treatment of patients after immune-mediated damage has already destroyed intrahepatic bile ducts. Second, progressive destruction of bile ducts by NSDC initiates secondary pathogenetic mechanisms caused by biliary obstruction and cholestasis, which independently are capable of progression to biliary cirrhosis[7]. Thus, at the time of diagnosis, both primary immunologic and secondary obstructive mechanisms of pathogenesis are concurrently involved in most patients with PBC. Third, the finding that one mouse monoclonal antibody produced by immunization with PDC-E2 reacted intensely with non-mitochondrial antigen in the apical cytoplasm of biliary epithelial cells in PBC suggested the possibility of molecular mimicry and an infectious etiology[8]. Recent findings that this mouse monoclonal antibody reacts avidly with linear decapeptide mimotopes and that immunization of rabbits with the mimotopes results in polyclonal antibodies that cross-react with the apical antigen in PBC biliary epithelial cells are consistent with the hypothesis that PBC is an infectious disease[9,10]. If PBC were an infectious rather than autoimmune disease, poor response to immunosuppressant medications would be expected.

IMMUNOSUPPRESSION IN PRIMARY BILIARY CIRRHOSIS

The goals of immunosuppression in PBC are to prevent or retard immuno-logic mechanisms of NSDC, periportal hepatitis and cytokine-induced portal fibrosis while minimizing morbidity and mortality associated with immuno-suppression. Primary and secondary end-points of immunosuppressive ther-apy, however, are difficult to define and measure given the heterogeneity of PBC patients entering therapeutic trials and the coexistence of both immuno-logic and biliary obstructive pathogenic mechanisms. Currently, a variety of medications are available or under investigation to suppress the activation and functions of immunologic cells[11] with different degrees of selectivity (Table 2). Unfortunately, long-term immunosuppression is associated with complications of drug toxicity, infection and malignancy. Over the past two

Table 2 Effects of immunosuppressive drugs on target tissues

Drug	Bone marrow	Granulocytes	Platelets	Resting T and B cells	Memory T and B cells	Activated T and B cells
Corticosteroids	0	0	+	+	+	+
Azathioprine	+	+	+	+	+	+
OKT3/OKT4	0	0	0	+	+	+
Cyclosporine	0	0	0	0	0	+
Tacrolimus	0	0	0	0	0	+
Mycophenolate	0	0	0	0	0	+
Sirolimus	0	0	0	0	0	+
Mizoribine	0	0	0	0	0	+
Gusperimus	0	0	0	0	0	+

Table 3 Immunosuppressant drugs without benefit in primary biliary cirrhosis

D-penicillamine
Azathioprine
Chlorambucil
Levamisole
Malotilate
Thalidomide?

decades, several immunosuppressant drugs have been tested in PBC without objective evidence of benefit (Table 3).

IMMUNOSUPPRESSIVE AGENTS: MECHANISMS AND POTENTIAL

The site of action of individual immunosuppressant agents is summarized in Figure 1. At the time of diagnosis, initiation of the immune response in PBC may have occurred years earlier; thus, the most plausible therapeutic strategies would be to: (a) prevent ongoing sensitization of new precursor T and B cells, and (b) inhibit proliferation and functions of established effector cells.

Corticosteroids

Corticosteroids, principally prednisone and prednisolone, have complex anti-inflammatory and immunosuppressive actions[12]. In humans, steroids decrease lymphocytes, monocytes, eosinophils, and basophils in peripheral blood as a result of redistribution from the intravascular space rather than lysis. Anti-inflammatory and immunosuppressive actions of glucocorticoids are directly linked by the steroid inhibition of leukocyte functions. Corticosteroids impact on diverse elements of the afferent and efferent limbs of the immune response. By suppressing monocyte secretion of IL-1 and TNF-α, they diminish the effectiveness of antigen presentation to T cells and the differentiation of B cells necessary for immunoglobulin secretion. In addition, they suppress IL-2 secretion by CD4 T cells required for clonal expansion of activated CD4 and CD8 T cells. Toxicities of long-term use include: fluid and electrolyte disturbances, hypertension, cataracts, glaucoma,

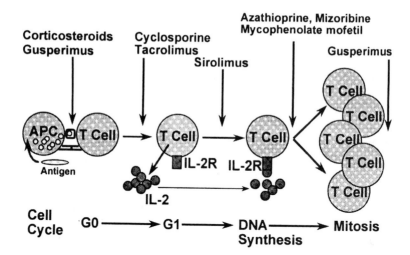

Figure 1 Specific sites of action of immunosuppressive agents during an immune response. See text for detailed description of the mechanism of action of each drug. Adapted from Reference 12.

osteoporosis, cutaneous atrophy, acne, bruising, poor wound healing, gastritis, glucose intolerance, emotional changes, impotence and amenorrhea. Although corticosteroids remain a controversial therapy in PBC, a three-year placebo-controlled trial indicated a beneficial response without significant acceleration of bone demineralization[13].

Azathioprine

Azathioprine, an antimetabolite prodrug of mercaptopurine, is converted into mercaptopurine-containing nucleotides that are incorporated into cellular DNA, inhibiting purine nucleotide synthesis and metabolism[12]. These effects prevent proliferation of rapidly dividing cells, such as T and B lymphocytes. Since its antiproliferative effect is non-specific, azathioprine is also myelosuppressive and reduces the quantities of circulating platelets, granuloctyes and monocytes. In addition to myelosuppression, azathioprine is occasionally hepatotoxic and is associated with an increased incidence of malignancies when used chronically. It is considered ineffective as mono-therapy for PBC[14].

Cyclosporine

Cyclosporine is a product of the fungus *Tolypocladium inflatum*[11,12]. A third-generation microemulsion formulation has been introduced to enhance absorption from the small bowel. Cyclosporine binds to intracytoplasmic cyclophilin receptors in CD4 T cells and inhibits calcineurin phosphatase (Figure 2). Calcineurin phosphatase activity is required for transcription factors involved in the activation of genes encoding IL-2, IL-3, IL-4, TNF-α, INF-γ and granulocyte-macrophage colony-stimulating factor (GM–CSF).

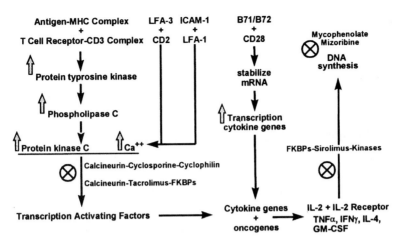

Figure 2 Intracellular events of T cell activation and sites of action of immunosuppressive agents. Adapted from Reference 11.

These genes and their translational products are critical for a T cell immune response. Cyclosporine also increases expression of transformation growth factor-beta (TGF-β) *in vitro*. Since TGF-β is a potent T cell suppressant cytokine[2], it may contribute to the immunosuppressive effects of cyclosporine. The principal toxicities of cyclosporine include: nephrotoxicity, neurotoxicity, hypertension, hypercholesterolemia, hirsutism, gynecomastia, gingival hyperplasia, lymphoproliferative disorders and rare hepatotoxicity. A long-term, randomized trial of 300 patients with PBC showed no benefit[15], and PBC has been reported to recur while on cyclosporine following orthotopic liver transplantation[16].

Tacrolimus (FK-506)

Tacrolimus is a macrolactam, produced by *Streptomyces tsukubeaensis*. Despite structural differences with cyclosporine, tacrolimus suppresses the immune response of CD4 T cells by a similar mechanism (Figure 2). Specifically, tacrolimus binds to cytoplasmic FK-binding proteins (FKBPs) within T cells[11,12]. The principal isoform responsible for immunosuppression is FKBP12. The association of tacrolimus–FKBP complexes with Ca^{2+}-dependent calcineurin–calmodulin complexes inhibits Ca^{2+}-dependent signal transduction following the Ca^{2+} influx triggered by T cell receptor activation. Transcription factors required for activation of cytokine genes are either direct or indirect substrates of calcineurin's serine–threonine phosphatase activity, which is inhibited by binding of tacrolimus–FKBP complexes with calcineurin. As with cyclosporine, tacrolimus decreases transcription of IL-2, IL-3, IL-4, IL-5, TNF-α, IFN-γ, and GM–CSF. In addition, tacrolimus also inhibits expression of IL-2 and IL-7 receptors on T cells. The principal toxicities of tacrolimus include: nephrotoxicity, neurotoxicity, hypertension, hypercholesterolemia, pancreatitis, glucose intolerance, gastrointestinal intolerance, allergic reactions, bone marrow suppression, alopecia, arthralgia and lymphoproliferative disorders. Tacrolimus has not been used in a long-term randomized controlled trial in PBC. Since its mechanism of immunosuppression is similar to cyclosporine, it is not expected to have great benefit as monotherapy. Moreover, recurrence of PBC during tacrolimus immunosuppression after orthotopic liver transplantation has been reported[16].

Mycophenolate mofetil

Mycophenolate mofetil is a prodrug hydrolyzed by liver esterases to produce mycophenolic acid. Mycophenolic acid is a non-competitive reversible inhibitor of inosine monophosphate dehydrogenase, the critical enzyme for *de novo* synthesis of purines required for proliferation of activated lymphocytes[17]. By inhibiting purine synthesis, mycophenolic acid prevents mixed lymphocyte reactions to alloantigens, the proliferative responses of both T and B cells to mitogens, cell surface expression of IL-2 receptors, HLA-DR and transferrin receptors, and Ig synthesis by T-cell independent activated B cells. It also interferes with glycosylation of adhesion molecules required for T cell activation and cytotoxic function. At high concentrations mycophenolic acid also inhibits IL-4- or IL-13-induced IgE synthesis. It has no effect on neutrophil chemotaxis or neutrophil production of superoxide, synthesis of IL-1β, IL-6 or TNF-α by monocytes, or IL-2, IL-4 and IL-13 production by lymphocytes. Toxicities are generally minor and include: diarrhea, abdominal pain, nausea and vomiting, leukopenia and anemia. Mycophenolate mofetil has not been studied in PBC, but its toxicity and ability to inhibit both T and B cell functions make it an attractive candidate.

Methotrexate

Methotrexate is an antimetabolite with both immunosuppressant and antiproliferative actions[18]. Its mechanisms of action include inhibition of dihydrofolate reductase and folate-dependent enzymes required for both *de novo* purine and thymidylate synthesis. Methotrexate has been extensively used for the treatment of psoriasis, refractory rheumatoid arthritis, chronic graft-versus-host disease and in many cancer chemotherapy regimens. Its principal toxicities include: bone marrow suppression, mucositis, alopecia, dermatitis, interstitial pneumonitis, nephrotoxicity, abortion, teratogenesis and hepatic fibrosis. Controlled trials of methotrexate monotherapy and combination therapy with ursodeoxycholic acid are ongoing.

Ursodeoxycholic acid

Ursodeoxycholic acid (UDCA) is an anticholestatic agent with weak immunosuppressive actions[19]. It is unequivocally beneficial in retarding progression of PBC regardless of disease severity[20]. In a recent report of its immunosuppressive potency, it was added to standard immunosuppression in 50 consecutive adult patients who had experienced one episode of acute rejection after liver transplantation. Absence of steroid-resistant rejection in

49 of the 50 suggested a beneficial effect[21]. However, a double-blind randomized trial[22] did not show reduction in incidence or severity of rejection. Design of future trials of immunosuppressants in PBC will most likely combine one or more drugs with UDCA.

Thalidomide

Thalidomide is a TNF antagonist useful in the treatment of steroid-resistant graft-versus-host disease[23]. In a randomized double-blind placebo-controlled trial in 18 patients with PBC, thalidomide did not improve liver tests or histology[24]. It is important to note that the dose was substantially less than that used to treat graft-versus-host disease. The principal adverse effects were sedation and fatigue.

INVESTIGATIONAL IMMUNOSUPPRESSIVE AGENTS

Sirolimus (rapamycin)

Sirolimus, an immunosuppressive agent isolated from the actinomycete *Streptomyces hygroscopicus*, is structurally related to tacrolimus[11]. After entry into cells, the portion of the macrolactam ring structure shared with tacrolimus binds to cytosolic FKBPs. Although sirolimus–FKBP complexes are necessary for biologic effects, the targets of these intracellular complexes are undefined. Sirolimus suppression of protein synthesis in T cells is possibly related to inhibition of the 79-kDa S6 kinase responsible for the protein synthetic activity of the S6 ribosomal protein. In contrast to cyclosporine and tacrolimus which block T cell progression from G0 to G1 (Figure 1), sirolimus prevents progression from G1 to S phase of the cell cycle. This may be due to reduced kinase activity of CDk2/cyclinE complex. Sirolimus does not alter early events of T cell activation and is not an effective inhibitor of cytokine synthesis. In contrast to cyclosporine or tacrolimus, sirolimus inhibits activation of T cells by IL-2, IL-4, IL-6 and anti-CD28 antibody. It also blocks lipopolysaccharide stimulation of B cell proliferation. Sirolimus inhibits Ca^{2+}-independent signaling in both T and B cells (Figure 2). The ability of sirolimus to block the mitogenic effects of cytokines, such as IL-2, makes it a candidate drug in PBC.

Mizoribine

Mizoribine is an imidazole nucleoside antibiotic produced by the fungus *Eupenicillium brefeldianum*[11]. Mizoribine is a prodrug that is phosphorylyzed by adenosine kinase to form mizoribine 5′-monophosphate, a competitive inhibitor of inosine monophosphate dehydrogenase and guanosine monophosphate synthetase. The active drug is not incorporated into either DNA or RNA and is dephosphorylated intracellularly by 5′-nucleotidase. Mizoribine immunosuppression is additive to that of either cyclosporine or tacrolimus and permits reduction of the dose of either drug when used in combination. Since it is also steroid-sparing, it may be useful in combination.

Gusperimus (deoxyspergualin)

Gusperimus is an analog of the parent drug spergualin isolated from *Bacillus laterosporus*[11]. Currently, it is produced by organic synthesis. The mechanisms of gusperimus functional inhibition of antigen-presenting cells and T and B cells are poorly understood. It appears to act at two independent stages: (a) alloantigen processing and presentation in the afferent limb of the immune response, and (b) inhibition of maturation and differentiated function of T and B cells in the effector limb. Gusperimus binding to Hsc70, a cytosolic protein of the heat shock protein family, may be involved in inhibition of antigen processing and presentation. It is postulated that gusperimus competes for the Hsc70 peptide-binding site and inhibits the processing of antigenic peptides necessary for presentation of MHC–alloantigen complexes to T cell receptors. Gusperimus inhibits differentiation of cytotoxic function in activated T cells by unknown mechanisms. It also prevents maturation of B cells stimulated with endotoxin or IFN-γ by interfering with nuclear transcription factor NFκB. Gusperimus also weakly inhibits proliferation in mixed lymphocyte reactions and reduces IL-2 receptor expression on both CD4 and CD8 T cells. However, it does not inhibit proliferation of T or B cells induced by most mitogens. Since gusperimus can inhibit differentiation of cytotoxic T cell function, it may be useful in reducing the impact of cytotoxic CD8 T cells mediating NSDC.

FUTURE DIRECTIONS

Further understanding of the immunopathogenesis of PBC is mandatory for future development of therapeutics. A key unresolved question is whether PBC is an infectious, rather than autoimmune, disease. If immunosuppression is found to be warranted in PBC, it will likely be administered as combination therapy and tailored to the histopathologic stage of disease. Thus, therapeutic trials will require enrollment of disproportionate numbers of patients with prefibrotic stages of disease.

References

1. Vierling JM. Primary biliary cirrhosis. In: Zakim D, Boyer TD (eds). Hepatology, 2nd Edn. Philadelphia: W.B. Saunders Co.; 1990:1158–205.
2. Vierling JM, Hu K I-Q. Immunologic mechanisms of hepatobiliary injury. In: Kaplowitz N (ed). Liver and Biliary Diseases, 2nd Edn. Baltimore, Maryland: Williams & Wilkins; 1996:55–87.
3. Que FG, Gores GJ. Cell death by apoptosis: basic concepts and disease relevance for the gastroenterologist. Gastroenterology 1996;110:1238–43.
4. Harada K, Van de Water J, Leung PS, *et al*. *In situ* nucleic acid hybridization of cytokines in primary biliary cirrhosis: predominance of the Th1 subset. Hepatology 1997;25:791–6.
5. Leung PS, Van de Water J, Coppel RL, Nakanuma Y, Munoz S, Gershwin ME. Molecular aspects and the pathological basis of primary biliary cirrhosis. J Autoimmun 1996;9:119–28.
6. Freilich BL, Hu K-Q, Vierling JM. Immunopathogenesis of autoimmune hepatobiliary diseases. Curr Opin Gastroenterol 1994;10:257–68.
7. Desmet V, Roskams T, Van Eyken P. Ductular reaction in the liver. Pathol Res Pract 1995;191:513–24.

8. Van de Water J, Turchany J, Leung PS, *et al.* Molecular mimicry in primary biliary cirrhosis: Evidence for biliary epithelial expression of a molecule cross-reactive with pyruvate dehydrogenase-E2. J Clin Invest 1993;91:2653–64.

9. Leung PS, Cha S, Joplin RE, *et al.* Inhibition of PDC-E2 human combinatorial autoantibodies by peptide mimotopes. J Autoimmun 1996;9:785–93.

10. Cha S, Leung PS, Van de Water J, *et al.* Random phage mimotopes recognized by monoclonal antibodies against the pyruvate dehydrogenase complex-E2 (PDC-E2). Proc Natl Acad Sci USA 1996;93:10949–54.

11. Morris RE. New immunosuppressive drugs. In: Busuttil RW, Klintmalm GB (eds). Transplantation of the Liver. Philadelphia, Pennsylvania: W.B. Saunders Co.; 1996:760–86.

12. Vierling JM. Immunology of hepatic allograft rejection. In: Maddrey WC, Sorrell MF (eds). Transplantation of the Liver, 2nd Edn. Norwalk, Connecticut: Appleton & Lange; 1995:367–98.

13. Mitchison HC, Palmer JM, Bassendine MF, Watson AJ, Record CO, James OF. A controlled trial of prednisolone treatment in primary biliary cirrhosis. Three-year results. J Hepatol 1992;15:336–44.

14. Christensen E, Neuberger J, Crowe J, *et al.* Beneficial effect of azathioprine and prediction of prognosis in primary biliary cirrhosis. Final results of an international trial. Gastroenterology 1985;89:1084–91.

15. Lombard M, Portman B. Neuberger J, *et al.* Cyclosporin A treatment in primary biliary cirrhosis: results of a long-term placebo controlled trial. Gastroenterology 1993;104:519–26.

16. Van de Water J, Gerson LB, Ferrell LD, *et al.* Immunohistochemical evidence of disease recurrence after liver transplantation for primary biliary cirrhosis. Hepatology 1996; 24:1079–84.

17. Sievers TM, Rossi SJ, Ghobrial RM, *et al.* Mycophenolate mofetil. Pharmacotherapy 1997;17:1178–97.

18. Peters LJ, Olsen NJ. Mechanisms of action of methotrexate. Bull Rheum Dis 1991;41:5–8.

19. Yoshikawa M, Tsujii T, Matsumura K, *et al.* Immunoregulatory effects of ursodeoxycholic acid on immune responses. Hepatology 1992;16:358–64.

20. Poupon RE, Lindor KD, Cauch-Dudek K, Dickson ER, Poupon R, Heathecote EJ. Combined analysis of randomized controlled trials of ursodeoxycholic acid in primary biliary cirrhosis. Gastroenterology 1997;113:884–90.

21. Clavien PA, Sharara AJ, Camargo CA, *et al.* Evidence that ursodeoxycholic acid prevents steroid-resistant rejection in adult liver transplantation. Clin Transplant 1996;10:658–62.

22. Pageaux GP, Blanc P, Perigault PF, *et al.* Failure of ursodeoxycholic acid to prevent acute cellular rejection after liver transplantation. J Hepatol 1995;23:119–22.

23. Vogelsang GB, Farmer ER, Hess AD, *et al.* Thalidomide for the treatment of chronic graft-versus-host disease. N Engl J Med 1992;326:1055–8.

24. McCormick PA, Scott F, Epstein O, Burroughs AK, Scheur PJ, McIntyre N. Thalidomide therapy for primary biliary cirrhosis: a double-blind placebo controlled pilot study. J Hepatol 1994;21:496–9.

15
Methotrexate and colchicine in the treatment of primary biliary cirrhosis

M. M. KAPLAN

Colchicine and methotrexate continue to be evaluated in the treatment of primary biliary cirrhosis (PBC). Although most prospective studies demonstrate that colchicine improves biochemical tests of liver function, albeit to a lesser degree than ursodiol, there is still no agreement concerning its effectiveness in this disease. The data on methotrexate are mixed. Some studies suggest efficacy and others do not. Results of studies to determine whether either colchicine or methotrexate has any additive effect to that of ursodeoxycholic acid (UDCA) are also at variance. In the author's experience both drugs have demonstrated efficacy when adequate doses are used. In addition, methotrexate has had additive effects to those of UDCA if given to patients who have responded incompletely or not at all to UDCA, and colchicine has been effective in a subgroup of patients who have responded incompletely to the combination of UDCA and methotrexate. There is no reason to give either drug to the patient who responds completely to UDCA.

COLCHICINE

Three double-blind studies performed more than a decade ago compared colchicine to placebo in the treatment of PBC[1-4]. All reported some efficacy and little toxicity. The mechanism of action of colchicine in PBC is uncertain but may include the modulation of local cytokine and autacoid production by chronically stimulated macrophages, monocytes and lymphocytes[5-7]. Colchicine also inhibits endothelial adhesiveness for neutrophils, diminishes the expression of L-selectins on neutrophil cell surfaces, and affects the activity of cytokines, such as interleukin-2 and tumor necrosis factor in patients with PBC[8].

In an initial study of 60 patients, the administration of colchicine, compared with placebo, was associated with significant improvements in serum alkaline phosphatase, alanine and aspartate aminotransferase, albumin, bilirubin and cholesterol at two years[1]. The likelihood of death due to liver-related causes after four years was significantly lower in the patients started on colchicine. The results of the other two studies were similar but not statistically significant[2,3]. There was no improvement in symptoms or histology in any study. When survival data were pooled and analyzed in these three studies, colchicine significantly prolonged survival compared to placebo (M. M. Kaplan, unpublished data). When data were analyzed after eight years in one of these studies, biochemical tests were still improved in the colchicine-treated patients but the survival benefit was lost[4].

A recent placebo-controlled prospective trial randomized 90 patients to colchicine, ursodeoxycholic acid (UDCA), or placebo[9,10]. The following results were noted. Pruritus was significantly decreased with both colchicine and UDCA. Colchicine improved biochemical tests significantly but modestly whereas UDCA decreased serum alkaline phosphatase and aminotransferase activities more than placebo or colchicine. Serum bilirubin levels fell only in those receiving UDCA. UDCA, but not colchicine, reduced ductular proliferation. The authors concluded that both drugs were more effective than placebo and that UDCA was superior to colchicine in the treatment of PBC[10]. In an ongoing prospective study comparing colchicine with methotrexate in 70 patients with PBC, colchicine significantly decreased serum levels of alkaline phosphatase and ALT but had no effect on serum bilirubin or albumin[11].

Ursodeoxycholic acid is the drug used most often to treat PBC and has recently been approved by the US Food and Drug Administration for this purpose. Because both UDCA and colchicine are safe and both demonstrate some efficacy, it would be useful to know whether there is added benefit in using the two together. Unfortunately, there are not yet enough data to be certain[12]. Results of studies thus far are at variance and many are published in abstract form[13–16]. In one completed study, Poupon et al. found no added benefit when UDCA alone was compared with UDCA plus colchicine in 74 patients who still had abnormal liver function tests, particularly serum alkaline phosphatase, after at least eight months of treatment with UDCA[17]. There was no improvement in symptoms, liver function tests, IgM levels, serum markers of fibrosis, or histologic features except for lobular inflammation. Patients receiving the combination did have a reduced rate of progression of esophageal varices but the difference was not significant. In a similar study Ikeda et al. reported just the opposite results[18]. Twenty-two patients who had been receiving UDCA, 600 mg per day, for 30 months were randomly assigned to colchicine, 1 mg per day, plus UDCA ($n = 10$) or UDCA alone. In the group receiving both drugs there was a significant improvement in serum bilirubin, alkaline phosphatase, ALT, AST, γ-glutamyltransferase and IgM. This improvement was most marked in patients who had responded incompletely to UDCA. There was no additional improvement in blood tests in those who received UDCA alone. In another smaller study, UDCA and colchicine also appeared to have synergistic effects when used together for 2 years in 12 patients[19]. Serum concentrations of alkaline phosphatase and bilirubin were lower after three months in patients treated with combination therapy compared with those who received only UDCA. Combination therapy also decreased piecemeal necrosis and portal inflammation in the 8 patients who had follow-up liver biopsies.

The data suggest that colchicine improves biochemical tests of liver function in PBC but to a lesser degree than does UDCA. It may improve itching but clearly does not improve fatigue or histology. It may slow the progression of PBC. More data are needed, particularly in patients who have not responded completely to UDCA, to determine if colchicine has any additive effects to those of UDCA.

METHOTREXATE

Methotrexate was first used to treat PBC in 1986 because of an initially unexpected but encouraging experience with this drug in several patients with primary sclerosing cholangitis, another cholestatic liver disease with some similarities to PBC[20,21]. In the low doses used to treat PBC (0.25 mg/kg body weight per week orally), methotrexate may act as an immunomodulatory and/or anti-inflammatory agent rather than as an antimetabolite[22-25].

Methotrexate was initially evaluated in nine symptomatic patients with PBC[26]. Serum alkaline phosphatase, alanine aminotransferase, aspartate aminotransferase, cholesterol and bilirubin all significantly decreased while serum albumin remained normal. Biochemical tests became normal in some patients after prolonged treatment for 24–60 months. Fatigue and/or itching improved or resolved in all 9 patients. Liver histology improved in 5 patients and stabilized in 4. The response to methotrexate was slower than that to UDCA and occurred over several years. Positive responses to methotrexate have been seen primarily in patients with precirrhotic PBC. Methotrexate has been of no benefit in patients with advanced cirrhosis or decompensated liver disease.

Most patients who received methotrexate exhibited a transient increase in aminotransferase levels 2 weeks to 8 months after starting the drug, followed by a decrease and subsequent return to normal. This transient elevation in aminotransferase activity appeared to be a predictor of a favorable response to methotrexate. Similar results have been reported by Bergasa et al. in 10 patients with PBC[27]. Liver function tests and symptoms improved. There was decreased inflammation in repeat liver biopsies but increased fibrosis.

Methotrexate has now been used to treat more than 80 patients with PBC at the New England Medical Center, either as sole therapy or in combination with UDCA and colchicine in those who either failed to respond to these agents or did so only partially. The results have been similar to our original experience. In a recent study, 13 of 14 patients who responded incompletely or not at all to UDCA and/or colchicine showed significant improvement in liver function tests as well as improvement in symptoms and histology when methotrexate and/or colchicine was added[28]. In 9 of these 14 patients, the addition of methotrexate to UDCA alone or to UDCA plus colchicine was associated with a significant improvement in biochemical tests of liver function. In 2 of them, improvement occurred when colchicine was added to UDCA plus methotrexate and, in 2, it was not possible to determine whether methotrexate or colchicine was responsible for the improvement. These 2 drugs were added within a month's time of each other in two patients who had failed to respond to UDCA and already had advanced PBC histologically, early stage IV. Similar results were obtained in a second study in which methotrexate was given to 8 patients who had responded only partially to UDCA[29]. The addition of methotrexate improved both symptoms and biochemical tests more completely than UDCA alone.

There are also negative studies with methotrexate in PBC[30–32]. Lindor et al. reported no added benefit in 32 patients who received methotrexate plus UDCA when this group was compared with patients who were part of an earlier study of UDCA alone[30]. Because biochemical tests may become normal or improve greatly in many patients receiving UDCA alone[33], it is possible that an additive effect of methotrexate was missed. In a recently published study of 25 patients, no added benefit was observed when methotrexate, 10 mg per week, plus UDCA, 500 mg per day, was compared with UDCA alone, also 500 mg per day[32]. Patients were followed for 48 weeks. The dose of methotrexate used, 10 mg per week, is lower than the dose which is usually effective, 0.25 mg (kg body weight)$^{-1}$ week^{-1} or 12.5–17.5 mg/week in most female patients. A similarly negative study was recently reported in a study of 60 patients in which methotrexate, 7.5 mg/week, was compared with placebo in patients followed for up to 59 months on methotrexate[31]. This is a lower dose of methotrexate than is usually effective in PBC and is the dose at which virtually all patients who have responded to methotrexate relapsed when I tried to find the lowest effective dose in methotrexate responders (M. M. Kaplan, unpublished data).

We have recently reported sustained remission in 5 women with well-established PBC, stage II–IV, all of whom were antimitochondrial antibody positive. These patients have now been on medical therapy for their PBC for up to 15 years and on methotrexate for 7–9 years[34]. All had florid bile duct lesions at onset, striking inflammation within portal triads and granulomas within the liver. Biochemical tests of liver function returned to normal, pruritus and fatigue remitted in all, and serial liver biopsies demonstrated progressive improvement with a fall in mean histologic stage from 2.5 to 1.0. After five years of treatment, liver biopsies in two patients were normal and showed no signs of PBC.

Although methotrexate has been well tolerated in most patients, its long-term safety and efficacy in PBC have not been determined. Methotrexate caused a serious but reversible interstitial pneumonitis in approximately 15% of patients with PBC in one study[35]. It was manifested by a nonproductive cough and dyspnea, and responded rapidly to cessation of methotrexate and administration of glucocorticoids. For reasons that are unclear the incidence of methotrexate pneumonitis has been very much less common in my PBC patients since this high occurrence more than five years ago.

At this time, methotrexate is best used in clinical studies or cautiously in individual patients with PBC who are not responding to therapy with UDCA and/or colchicine and are clinically worsening. Early treatment of symptomatic patients is important because no medical therapy is likely to be helpful once cirrhosis and signs of liver failure have developed.

There is general agreement that PBC is a progressive disease in most patients. It eventually becomes irreversible, and therefore untreatable, at about the time that cirrhosis develops. In my experience, the risk-to-benefit ratio of drugs such as colchicine, UDCA, and methotrexate is better than that of no treatment with the eventual development of liver failure and the need for liver transplantation. In addition to the risks associated with major surgery, patients who survive liver transplantation face a lifetime of treatment with a combination of drugs including potent immunosuppressive drugs. Moreover, in my experience some patients with PBC may go into sustained remission if treated with UDCA, colchicine, and methotrexate, sometimes if used alone but more often when they are used in combination.

References

1. Kaplan MM, Alling DW, Zimmerman HJ, et al. A prospective trial of colchicine for primary biliary cirrhosis. N Engl J Med 1986;315:1448–54.
2. Warnes TW, Smith A, Lee FI, Haboubi NY, Johnson PJ, Hunt L. A controlled trial of colchicine in primary biliary cirrhosis. J Hepatol 1987;5:1–7.
3. Bodenheimer H Jr, Schaffner F, Pezzullo J. Evaluation of colchicine therapy in primary biliary cirrhosis. Gastroenterology 1988;95:124–9.
4. Zifroni A, Schaffner F. Long-term follow-up of patients with primary biliary cirrhosis on colchicine therapy. Hepatology 1991;14:990–3.
5. Wangoo A, Haynes AR, Sutcliffe SP, et al. Modulation of platelet derived growth factor B mRNA abundance in macrophages by colchicine and dibutyryl-c AMP. Mol Pharmacol 1992;42:584–9.
6. Kershenobich D, Rojkind M, Quiroga A, Alcocer-Varela J. Effect of colchicine on lymphocyte and monocyte function and its relation to fibroblast proliferation in primary biliary cirrhosis. Hepatology 1990;11:205–9.
7. Miller LC, Kaplan MM. Serum interleukin-2 and tumor necrosis factor-alpha in primary biliary cirrhosis. Am J Gastroenterol 1992;87:465–70.
8. Cronstein BN, Molad Y, Reibman J, Balakhane E, Levin RI, Weissmann G. Colchicine alters the quantitative and qualitative display of selectins on endothelial cells and neutrophils. J Clin Invest 1995;96:994–1002.
9. Miettinen TL, Farkkila M, Vuoristo M, et al. Serum cholestanol, cholesterol precursors, and plant sterols during placebo-controlled treatment of primary biliary cirrhosis with ursodeoxycholic acid or colchicine. Hepatology 1995;21:1261–8.
10. Vuoristo M, Farkkila M, Karvonen AL, et al. A placebo-controlled trial of primary biliary cirrhosis treatment with colchicine and ursodeoxycholic acid. Gastroenterology 1995;108:1470–8.
11. Kaplan M, Schmid C, McKusick A, Provenzale D, Sharma A, Sepe T. Double-blind trial of methotrexate (MTX) versus colchicine (COLCH) in primary biliary cirrhosis. Hepatology 1993;18:176A.
12. Lindor KD. Colchicine and ursodeoxycholic acid for primary biliary cirrhosis. Gastroenterology 1995;108:1592–4.
13. Bobadilla J, Vargas F, Dehasa M, et al. Colchicine and ursodiol in the treatment of primary biliary cirrhosis (abstract). Hepatology 1994;20:332A.
14. Goddard CJR, Hunt L, Smith A, Fallowfield G, Rowqan B, Warnes TW. A trial of ursodeoxycholic acid (UDCA) and colchicine in primary biliary cirrhosis (PBC) (abstract). Hepatology 1994;20:151A.
15. Almassio P, Provenzano G, Battezatti PM, et al. The Italian multicentre randomized controlled trial of ursodeoxycholic acid versus ursodeoxycholic acid plus colchicine in symptomatic primary biliary cirrhosis (abstract). Hepatology 1994;20:267A.

16. Poupon RE, Niard AM, Huet PM, *et al.* A randomized trial comparing the combination ursodeoxycholic acid (UDCA) and colchicine to ursodeoxycholic acid alone in primary biliary cirrhosis (abstract). Hepatology 1994;20:151A.
17. Poupon RE, Huet M, Poupon R, *et al.* A randomized trial comparing colchicine and ursodeoxycholic acid combination to ursodeoxycholic acid in primary biliary cirrhosis. Hepatology 1996;24:1098–103.
18. Ikeda T, Tozuka S, Noguchi O, *et al.* Effects of additional administration of colchicine in ursodeoxycholic acid-treated patients with primary biliary cirrhosis: a prospective randomized study. J Hepatol 1996;24:88–94.
19. Shibata J, Fujiyama S, Honda Y, Sato T. Combination therapy with ursodeoxycholic acid and colchicine for primary biliary cirrhosis. J Gastroenterol Hepatol 1992;7:277–82.
20. Kaplan MM, Arora S, Pincus SH. Primary sclerosing cholangitis and low dose oral pulse methotrexate. Ann Intern Med 1987;106:231–5.
21. Wiesner RH, LaRusso NF, Ludwig J, Dickson ER. Comparison of the clinicopathologic features of primary sclerosing cholangitis and primary biliary cirrhosis. Gastroenterology 1985;88:108–14.
22. Cronstein BN, Naime D, Ostad E. The antiinflammatory mechanism of methotrexate. Increased adenosine release at inflamed sites diminishes leukocyte accumulation in an in vivo model of inflammation. J Clin Invest 1993;92:2675–82.
23. Weinstein GD, Jeffes E, McCullough JL. Cytotoxic and immunologic effects of methotrexate in psoriasis. J Invest Dermatol 1990;95:49S–52S.
24. Segal R, Yaron M, Tartakovsky B. Methotrexate: mechanisms of action in rheumatoid arthritis. Semin Arthritis Rheum 1990;20:190–9.
25. Suarez CR, Pickett WC, Beu DH, *et al.* Effect of low dose methotrexate neutrophil chemotaxis induced by leukotriene B4 and complement c5a. J Rheumatol 1987;14:9–11.
26. Kaplan MM, Knox TA. Treatment of primary biliary cirrhosis with low-dose weekly methotrexate. Gastroenterology 1991;101:1332–8.
27. Bergasa NV, Jones A, Kleiner DE, *et al.* Pilot study of low dose oral methotrexate treatment for primary biliary cirrhosis. Am J Gastroenterol 1996;91:295–9.
28. Bonis PA, Kaplan MM. The effects of colchicine and methotrexate are additive to ursodeoxycholic acid for patients with primary biliary cirrhosis (PBC) who have responded incompletely to ursodeoxycholic acid. Hepatology 1997;26:438A.
29. Buscher HP, Zietzschmann Y, Gerok W. Positive responses to methotrexate and ursodeoxycholic acid in patients with primary biliary cirrhosis responding insufficiently to ursodeoxycholic acid. J Hepatol 1993;18:9–14.
30. Lindor KD, Dickson ER, Jorgensen RA, *et al.* The combination of ursodeoxycholic acid and methotrexate for patients with primary biliary cirrhosis: the results of a pilot study. Hepatology 1995;22:1158–62.
31. Hendrickse M, Rigney E, Giaffer MH, *et al.* Low-dose methotrexate in primary biliary cirrhosis: long-term results of a placebo-controlled trial. Hepatology 1997;26:248A.
32. Gonzalez-Koch A, Brahm J, Antezana C, Smok G, Cumsille MA. The combination of ursodeoxycholic acid and methotrexate for primary biliary cirrhosis is not better then ursodeoxycholic acid alone. Am J Gastroenterol 1997;27:143–9.
33. Jorgensen RA, Dickson ER, Hofmann AF, Rossi SS, Lindor KD. Characterisation of patients with a complete biochemical response to ursodeoxycholic acid. Gut 1995;36:935–8.
34. Kaplan M, DeLellis R, Wolfe H. Sustained biochemical and histological remission of primary biliary cirrhosis in response to medical treatment. Ann Intern Med 1997;126:682–8.
35. Sharma A, Provenzale D, McKusick A, Kaplan MM. Interstitial pneumonitis after low-dose methotrexate therapy in primary biliary cirrhosis. Gastroenterology 1994;107:266–70.

16
Corticosteroids in PBC

H. R. van BUUREN

Primary biliary cirrhosis (PBC) is a chronic and usually slowly progressive cholestatic liver disease of unknown etiology. The disease has features indicating an (auto)immune-mediated disorder and attempts at finding effective medical therapy have largely been focused on drugs with immunomodulating potential. Among the numerous agents that have been evaluated for therapy[1], corticosteroids were not only the first to be used, but also the first to be considered unsuitable[2,3]. The early negative experience with steroids has subsequently prevented adequate exploration of their therapeutic potential for decades. During recent years, however, recognition of the partial efficacy of bile acid treatment, a better understanding of the dangers associated with steroid treatment, the introduction of improved tools for monitoring bone mass and the development of effective therapy for treating bone loss have all contributed to a renewed interest in corticosteroids as therapeutic agents in PBC.

EARLY EXPERIENCE

In 1960, Hoffbauer[2] reported his observations that were made on a group of 25 PBC patients during a 12-year period. At presentation, all but 4 were icteric and, during the period of observation, the mortality was 80%. Two patients received a trial with ACTH and 4 were treated with prednisone. Two patients were given a dose of 20 mg/day for 10–12 weeks; in one of these patients, vertebral compression fractures were noted after 10 weeks. No information was provided with respect to the dose or duration of treatment for the other patients. Obvious beneficial treatment effects were not observed.

In 1966, Howat et al.[3] reported their experience with 14 patients studied over a 14-year period. All patients were icteric at presentation. Eight were treated with cortisone, with doses ranging from 37.5 mg to 300 mg/day, and/or prednisone/prednisolone with doses that varied from 10 to 60 mg/day. In 5 of the 9 patients, aggravation of osteoporosis and bone fractures were observed. In addition, disseminated tuberculosis, peptic ulceration, suppurative otitis media, pneumonia and steroid cataracts were observed in one patient each. During the period of observation, 9/14 patients died. The authors concluded that "corticosteroids given in the terminal stages of primary biliary cirrhosis neither influence the clinical features nor the fatal outcome of the disease. When given in the earlier phases ... not only is itching relieved but clinical and biochemical improvement may ensue. Withdrawal of corticosteroids leads to relapse. The complications which accompany prolonged treatment by corticosteroids are so grave as to prohibit their use in primary biliary cirrhosis." It is obvious that nearly all patients in these series had far advanced, if not preterminal, disease and were *a priori* very unlikely to benefit from any medical therapy. A balanced judgement with respect to the usefulness of corticosteroids in PBC is further hampered by the uncontrolled character of the observations and the non-standardized, usually high, corticosteroid doses and the variable duration of treatment. Nevertheless, during subsequent decades, these reports dominated the medical attitude towards corticosteroids for PBC.

RECENT EXPERIENCE

Despite the reported negative experience with steroids in the sixties, some hepatologists continued to use corticosteroids, but this was only in occasional patients and not in the context of properly executed studies. It was not until 1989 that the preliminary results of a first randomized controlled trial were reported[4]. Since then, 2 more randomized controlled trials of corticosteroids in PBC have been performed. Although all these studies can be regarded as pilot investigations, the cumulative experience derived from these trials now allows a more balanced view with respect to the benefit–risk ratio of corticosteroids in PBC.

THE NEWCASTLE PREDNISOLONE TRIAL

In 1989, the Newcastle group reported the 1-year results of the first randomized controlled trial of prednisolone in PBC[4]. In 1992, a second paper reported the final, 3-year results of this pioneer study[5]. Thirty-six patients were included: 19 received prednisolone, initially 30 mg/day, tapered off to 10 mg within 8 weeks, and 17 received placebo. At entry, the mean serum bilirubin was elevated to 2 times the upper limit of normal and 8 patients had values over 60 μmol/L; 39% of patients had cirrhosis. In the steroid group, 7 patients had events possibly attributable to treatment: 2 had duodenal ulcers, 1 diabetes mellitus, 1 panophthalmitis, 1 esophageal reflux and 1 small furuncles. A mildly Cushingoid appearance was noted in 9 cases. In the placebo group, 1 patient underwent ulcer surgery, 1 had acute pancreatitis and 1 vaginal candidiasis. Median weight gain was 2 kg among the placebo survivors and 3 kg among the prednisolone survivors. Although bone densitometry values of the forearm and femur were in general lower in the corticosteroid group, these differences were not statistically significant at 3 years. No vertebral collapse was seen. At 3 years, in the prednisolone group, symptoms were improved and alkaline phosphatase, IgM and IgG were significantly lower compared with the placebo group, whereas the trend favored corticosteroid treatment for all other liver blood tests. In the placebo group, appearance of cirrhosis ($n = 4$) was more common than in the steroid group ($n = 1$). The authors made an assessment of overall hepatic function; the individual components of this score were hepatic mortality, doubling of serum bilirubin, fall in albumin > 6 g/L, new symptoms of portal hypertension and new appearance of cirrhosis. Four patients taking steroids showed progression according to any of these features compared with 11 placebo treated patients ($p < 0.01$). The author's impression was that patients with early disease were more likely to benefit than patients with advanced disease.

THE GERMAN PREDNISOLONE–UDCA TRIAL

In 1985, Ulrich Leuschner *et al.* were the first to observe positive effects of ursodeoxycholic acid (UDCA) treatment on liver function tests in patients with PBC[6]. Their subsequent long-term observations[7] indicated that UDCA was effective in delaying disease progression but did not lead to complete inactivation of the disease. This prompted this group to carry out a 9-month randomized trial, in 30 previously untreated patients, to assess whether the addition of an immunosuppressive agent to UDCA could further improve therapeutic results. Treatment with prednisolone, 10 mg/day, and UDCA, $10 \text{ mg kg}^{-1} \text{ day}^{-1}$ (15 patients) was compared with monotherapy with UDCA plus placebo. Patients with cirrhosis were excluded; 23/30 patients had PBC histological stage I or II and serum bilirubin was normal in all. Three of the 15 patients treated with prednisolone developed features of Cushing's syndrome or hirsutism; no other adverse effects were observed. Bone densitometry of the lumbar spine revealed no significant changes in either treatment group. In both groups laboratory parameters improved significantly and no major differences between the groups were found. The most important finding in this trial was that liver histology improved significantly in the group treated with UDCA–prednisolone. Analysis of cumulative scores for 7 histological parameters showed mild or marked deterioration in 5/14 evaluated patients in the UDCA monotherapy group vs. only 1 in the combined-treatment group. Histological improvement was not established in the UDCA group whereas 7/15 patients receiving combined therapy improved ($p < 0.003$).

THE DUTCH PREDNISONE/AZATHIOPRINE/UDCA TRIAL

In a previous study by the Dutch Multicentre PBC Study Group, complete biochemical normalization was obtained in 11% of patients treated with UDCA; in at most 4% of the patients, clinical, biochemical, and histological remission was achieved[8]. Anecdotal experience in 7 patients treated in Rotterdam suggested that corticosteroids, azathioprine and UDCA had an additive therapeutic effect on symptoms and biochemical and immunological indices of the disease[9]. Azathioprine has a well-known corticosteroid-sparing effect; for several decades it has been successfully used for treating auto-immune hepatitis, either in combination with corticosteroids or as a single agent for maintaining remission. In PBC, azathioprine treatment was associ-

Table 1 Clinical events/potential adverse treatment effects in a trial comparing UDCA + prednisone + azathiopine with UDCA + matching placebos

	UDCA + prednisone + azathioprine	*UDCA + placebo*
Weight gain		
> 2.5 kg	10	4
> 5 kg	8	1
Cushingoid appearance	8	0
Hypertension*	4	1
Ecchymosis	3	3
Hirsutism	2	0
NIDDM	1	2
Cytopenia†	2	2
Infections	1	7
Gastrointestinal complaints	7	3
Peritonitis (laparotomy)	0	1
Partial portomesenterial thrombosis	1	0
Traumatic vertebral fracture	0	1
Edema	2	0
Angina pectoris	0	1

* Diastolic pressure increased to ≥ 95 mmHg or by ≥ 20 mmHg on 2 consecutive visits.
† WBC $< 2.5 \times 10^9$/L and/or platelets $< 70 \times 10^9$/L.

ated with mild improvement in survival in a large previous trial[10] and corticosteroids were shown to be of benefit in delaying disease progression[5].

Based on these data, a 1-year controlled trial was performed in the Netherlands to assess the potential benefits and risks of combined UDCA, prednisone and azathioprine treatment. Fifty patients entered a multicenter, double-blind controlled trial comparing UDCA ($10 \, mg \, kg^{-1} \, day^{-1}$) + prednisone (10 mg/day) + azathioprine (50 mg/day) with UDCA + matching placebos. Prednisone was started at 30 mg/day and the dose was reduced at monthly intervals by 10 mg until the maintenance dose of 10 mg/day was achieved. In addition, 26 patients were treated with etidronate–calcium and 24 patients, all patients from two centers, were included in a trial evaluating etidronate–calcium vs. calcium alone. All patients had been treated with UDCA $10 \, mg \, kg^{-1} \, day^{-1}$ for at least 1 year. Patients with decompensated disease, defined as Child–Pugh score > 6, were excluded.

Patients were well matched for baseline characteristics. The mean age was 52 years; the mean serum bilirubin was normal; 36% of patients had histological stage I or II and 22% stage IV. Table 1 lists the clinical events/potential adverse treatment effects that were observed during the study. Weight gain, Cushingoid face and increase in blood pressure were more frequently observed in the patients treated with steroids, usually shortly after the initiation of therapy with relatively high prednisone doses. There was no evidence that other problems were more frequent in the corticosteroid group; in particular there was no increased incidence of infections, cytopenia, diabetes mellitus or fractures.

Pruritus improved to some extent, although significantly only in the 'triple' treatment group. Compared with the group treated with UDCA alone,

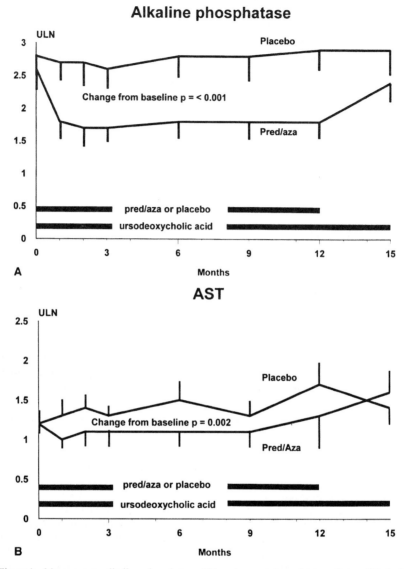

Figure 1 Mean serum alkaline phosphatase (A) and aspartate aminotransferase (B) during 1 year of UDCA + prednisone/azathioprine vs. UDCA + placebo and after 3 months of prednisone/azathioprine withdrawal. Data are expressed as multiples of the upper limit of normal (ULN). Error bars indicate standard errors.

serum alkaline phosphatase, ASAT, ALAT and IgM significantly decreased in the combined treatment group. After withdrawing prednisone and azathio-prine, this effect disappeared within 3 months (Figure 1). Liver biopsy was performed at entry and after 1 year. Detailed histological analysis showed significant improvements for the combined treatment group, in particular

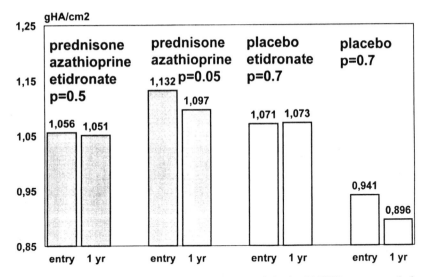

Figure 2 Mean values for lumbar (L2–L4) bone mineral density (DEXA) at entry and after 1 year. All patients were treated with calcium carbonate 500 mg/day.

in portal and lobular infiltrate. Differences between both groups were not significant. Evaluation of lumbar bone mass density using DEXA revealed no major differences between both groups. No changes in bone mass were observed for patients who had been treated with etidronate–calcium. Prednisone treated patients who had been treated with calcium alone showed a slight but significant fall in bone mass after one year. As expected, bone mass in placebo-treated patients was also lower after one year but changes were not significant (Figure 2).

CORTICOSTEROIDS AND METABOLIC BONE DISEASE

Corticosteroids may exacerbate the tendency to osteoporosis that complicates PBC. To what extent do steroids have a negative effect? As already discussed, high doses of corticosteroids given to patients with advanced disease may lead to serious osteoporosis and skeletal fractures[2,3]. In the Newcastle prednisolone trial[5], however, fractures were not observed and no significant differences in bone mass were found after 3 years between patients treated with corticosteroids and placebo-treated patients. A previous study from Rotterdam showed that, in general, bone loss in PBC was only moderate and related to the histological stage whereas no clinically important negative effect of corticosteroids on bone mass was observed[11]. Other studies have also been unable to document a clear deleterious effect of low-dose corticosteroids on the prevalence of skeletal fractures and bone density in patients with[12,13] and without liver disease[14]. In a small 1-year controlled pilot study, we assessed whether the bisphosphonate etidronate could reduce bone loss during corticosteroid treatment[15]. After one year, no significant changes in the mean lumbar bone mineral density in patients treated with etidronate–calcium were observed, in contrast to patients treated with calcium alone. The differences between both groups were significant. This finding is in agreement with studies in patients using corticosteroids for other (non-hepatic) diseases that showed prevention of bone loss by the use of bisphosphonates[16–21]. All studies have found this therapy to be safe.

DISCUSSION

Three randomized controlled trials have shown that corticosteroids, either as monotherapy or combined with UDCA, exert favorable treatment effects in PBC. Currently available data suggest that corticosteroids, like UDCA, are partially effective and do not seem able to induce clinical or biochemical remission in most patients. Corticosteroids have a number of potential adverse effects. The available data demonstrate that the risks should not be exaggerated. In the Dutch trial, weight gain and hypertension, in particular, seemed to be associated with the initial high prednisone dosage, and, as indicated by the experience of others, probably can be largely prevented by omitting high induction doses. In the past, the problem of corticosteroid-associated bone loss has been the major reason to abandon steroid treatment in PBC. Again, there are now several studies indicating that the negative effects of low-dose corticosteroid treatment on bone mass are not of major importance. Thus, with close attention to adequate dietary intake of calcium, vitamin D status and surveillance of bone mass, there is no major obstacle to using corticosteroids. Among the treatment options now available for treating osteoporosis or osteopenia, bisphosphonates may be the most attractive. The availability of these agents may further diminish fears for corticosteroids.

Interestingly, a controlled trial is now being performed by the Leuschner group with budesonide. The results are awaited with much interest since budesonide treatment may be associated with fewer adverse effects.

A favorable effect of corticosteroids on the long-term course of PBC is still insufficiently documented and further proof of their therapeutic significance is needed. The reported effects of monotherapies for PBC are limited and, therefore, it seems logical to concentrate on combinations of drugs that have been shown to be of some benefit[22]. In PBC, both immunological mechanisms and bile acid toxicity contribute to the chronic inflammatory hepatobiliary damage. Therefore, at least in theory, it seems attractive to combine drugs with different modes of action. Also, a combined treatment regimen may allow the use of relatively low doses of the individual drugs. Obviously, when long-term treatment is considered, the aspect of long-term safety is of primary importance. Based on these principles a European trial is now being prepared to assess the long-term effectiveness of UDCA combined with low-dose prednisolone–azathioprine.

References

1. Wiesner RH, Grambsch PM, Lindor KD, Ludwig J, Dickson ER. Clinical and statistical analyses of new and evolving therapies for primary biliary cirrhosis. Hepatology 1988;8:668–76.

2. Hoffbauer FW. Primary biliary cirrhosis. Observations on the natural course of the disease in 25 women. Am J Dig Dis 1960;5:348–83.
3. Howat HT, Ralston AJ, Varley H, Wilson JA. The late results of long-term treatment of primary biliary cirrhosis by corticosteroids. Rev Int Hepatol 1966;16:227–38.
4. Mitchison HC, Bassendine MF, Malcolm AJ, Watson AJ, Record CO, James OF. A pilot, double-blind, controlled 1-year trial of prednisolone treatment in primary biliary cirrhosis: hepatic improvement but greater bone loss. Hepatology 1989;10:420–9.
5. Mitchison HC, Palmer JM, Bassendine MF, Watson AJ, Record CO, James OF. A controlled trial of prednisolone treatment in primary biliary cirrhosis. Three-year results. J Hepatol 1992;15:336–44.
6. David R, Kurtz W, Strohm W, Leuschner U. Die wirkung von Ursodeoxycholsaure bei chronische leberkrankheiten. Eine Pilotstudie. Z Gastroenterol 1985;23:420(abstract).
7. Leuschner U, Guldutuna S, Imhof M, Hubner K, Benjaminov A, Leuschner M. Effects of ursodeoxycholic acid after 4 to 12 years of therapy in early and late stages of primary biliary cirrhosis. J Hepatol 1994;21:624–33.
8. Wolfhagen FH, van Buuren HR, Schalm SW, et al. Can ursodeoxycholic acid induce disease remission in primary biliary cirrhosis? The Dutch Multicentre PBC Study Group (letter). J Hepatol 1995;22:381.
9. Wolfhagen FH, van Buuren HR, Schalm SW. Combined treatment with ursodeoxycholic acid and prednisone in primary biliary cirrhosis. Neth J Med 1994;44:84–90.
10. Christensen E, Neuberger J, Crowe J et al. Beneficial effect of azathioprine and prediction of prognosis in primary biliary cirrhosis. Final results of an international trial. Gastroenterology 1985;89:1084–91.
11. Van Berkum FN, Beukers R, Birkenhager JC, Kooij PP, Schalm SW, Pols HA. Bone mass in women with primary biliary cirrhosis: the relation with histological stage and use of glucocorticoids. Gastroenterology 1990;99:1134–9.
12. Clements D, Compston JE, Rhodes J, Evans WD, Smith PM. Low-dose corticosteroids in chronic active hepatitis do not adversely affect spinal bone. Eur J Gastroenterol Hepatol 1993;5:543–7.
13. Diamond T, Stiel D, Lunzer M, Wilkinson M, Roche J, Posen S. Osteoporosis and skeletal fractures in chronic liver disease. Gut 1990;31:82–7.
14. Sambrook PN, Eisman JA, Yeates MG, Pocock NA, Eberl S, Champion GD. Osteoporosis in rheumatoid arthritis: safety of low dose corticosteroids. Ann Rheum Dis 1986;45:950–3.
15. Wolfhagen FHJ, van Buuren HR, den Ouden JW, et al. Cyclical etidronate in the prevention of bone loss in corticosteroid-treated primary biliary cirrhosis. J Hepatol 1997;26:325–30.
16. Reid IR, King AR, Alexander CJ, Ibbertson HK. Prevention of steroid-induced osteoporosis with (3-amino-1-hydroxypropylidene)-1,1-bisphosphonate (APD). Lancet 1988;1:143–6.
17. Adachi J, Cranney A, Goldsmith CH, et al. Intermittent cyclic therapy with etidronate in the prevention of corticosteroid induced bone loss. J Rheumatol 1994;21:1922–6.
18. Adachi JD, Bensen WG, Brown J, et al. Intermittent etidronate therapy to prevent corticosteroid-induced osteoporosis. N Engl J Med 1997;337:382–7.
19. Mulder H, Struys A. Intermittent cyclical etidronate in the prevention of corticosteroid-induced bone loss. Br J Rheumatol 1994;33:348–50.
20. Diamond T, McGuigan L, Barbagallo S, Bryant C. Cyclical etidronate plus ergocalciferol prevents glucocorticoid-induced bone loss in postmenopausal women. Am J Med 1995;98:459–63.
21. Struys A, Snelder AA, Mulder H. Cyclical etidronate reverses bone loss of the spine and proximal femur in patients with established corticosteroid-induced osteoporosis [see comments]. Am J Med 1995;99:235–42.
22. Kaplan MM. New strategies needed for treatment of primary biliary cirrhosis? Gastroenterology 1993;104:651–3.

17
Ursodeoxycholic acid treatment of primary biliary cirrhosis: potential mechanisms of action

G. PAUMGARTNER

During the past decade, there has been considerable progress in the treatment of chronic cholestatic liver diseases. Ursodeoxycholic acid has emerged as a safe and effective drug for the treatment of primary biliary cirrhosis. At present, it is the only treatment of primary biliary cirrhosis which not only improves serum liver tests[1-5] and certain histological features[2,5], but also prolongs survival free of liver transplantation[6,7]. A combined analysis[7] of three large randomized controlled trials of ursodeoxycholic acid in primary biliary cirrhosis from France[2], the United States[4] and Canada[3] included 548 patients who were randomized to receive either ursodeoxycholic acid or placebo. Patients treated with ursodeoxycholic acid had significantly improved survival free of liver transplantation. The effect on survival was most pronounced in the subgroup of high-risk patients with a serum bilirubin greater than 3.5 mg/dl. Since, in the French study and in the Canadian study, patients on placebo were offered ursodeoxycholic acid after two years, the true effect of ursodeoxycholic acid treatment on survival is probably greater than demonstrated in the combined analysis.

The mechanisms underlying the beneficial effects of ursodeoxycholic acid in primary biliary cirrhosis are still ill defined. In the following, I shall discuss three potential mechanisms of action of ursodeoxycholic acid:

(a) Protection of hepatocellular and cholangiocellular membranes against the detergent effects of hydrophobic bile acids;
(b) Stimulation of biliary secretion of endogenous hydrophobic bile acids and other cholephils;
(c) Reduction of MHC expression.

PROTECTION OF CELL MEMBRANES BY URSODEOXYCHOLIC ACID

Bile acids are biological detergents which, under pathological conditions, may injure hepatocellular and cholangiocellular membranes. The detergency

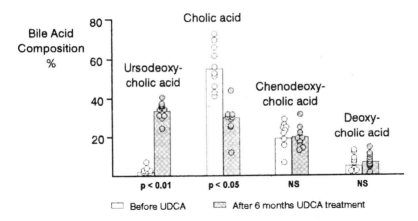

Figure 1 Relative proportions of the major conjugated bile acids (expressed as percentage of total conjugated bile acids) in the bile of patients with primary biliary cirrhosis before and after (shaded) six months of ursodeoxycholic acid (UDCA) treatment. Modified after Crosignani et al.[9]

of bile acids increases with increasing relative hydrophobicity as estimated by reverse-phase high-pressure liquid chromatography[8]. Endogenous hydrophobic bile acids may enhance the bile duct lesion in primary biliary cirrhosis and may, therefore, contribute to the pathogenesis of liver injury in cholestatic liver diseases by dissolving membrane lipids or stripping key hydrophobic proteins off the outer leaflet of the canalicular membrane of the hepatocyte or the apical membrane of the cholangiocyte.

The injurious effects of bile acids are aggravated by the fact that cholestasis causes retention of hydrophobic bile acids and other potentially toxic cholephils which may lead to liver cell injury, apoptosis and liver cell necrosis. As a consequence, liver fibrosis and cirrhosis may develop. It has been postulated that replacement of hydrophobic bile acids by a more hydrophilic bile acid, such as ursodeoxycholic acid, might be beneficial in this situation. The cytotoxic potential of bile acids is related to their relative hydrophobicity which decreases in the order taurodeoxycholic > taurochenodeoxycholic acid > taurocholic acid > tauroursodeoxycholic acid[8]. It has therefore been postulated that replacement of the more hydrophobic bile acids, chenodeoxycholic acid and deoxycholic acid, by ursodeoxycholic acid, a hydrophilic less-detergent and less-cytotoxic bile acid, might be beneficial in chronic cholestasis.

Under ursodeoxycholic acid treatment, the biliary bile acid composition becomes enriched with ursodeoxycholic acid[9]. After six months of ursodeoxycholic acid treatment of patients with primary biliary cirrhosis, ursodeoxycholic acid in bile increases to nearly 40% of total bile acids (Figure 1), rendering the bile acid composition less detergent. This may reduce bile acid injury at the site of the bile duct lesion in primary biliary cirrhosis. Heuman et al.[10] have shown that the physicochemical disruptive effects of bile acids towards membranes are a function of both concentration and hydrophobicity. As an index of canalicular disruption the solubilization of the structural canalicular ectoenzyme alkaline phosphatase under various *in-vitro* conditions was studied[11]. The hydrophobic bile acid taurodeoxycholic acid caused a release of alkaline phosphatase from the canalicular membranes in a concentration-dependent manner. This effect was inhibited by the addition of tauroursodeoxycholic acid. The magnitudes of these disruptive and protective effects were dependent not only upon the concentrations of the bile acids, but also on the concentrations of lipids. Lecithin:cholesterol vesicles at concentrations found in bile markedly reduced the disruption of canalicular membranes by taurodeoxycholic acid. This confirms previous findings that phospholipids can reduce the cytolytic effects of bile acids towards hepatocytes[12]. The concentrations of bile acids employed in these studies are those of bile and are, therefore, relevant for assessing the effects which ursodeoxycholic acid treatment exerts at the level of the bile ducts.

The mdr2 knock out mouse, in which phospholipids in bile are practically absent and cholesterol concentrations in bile are reduced, has been an excellent model to study the protective effects of ursodeoxycholic acid[13]. Normally, the cholangiocytes are protected against the detergent effects of bile acids by phospholipids, which are secreted by the mdr2 P-glycoprotein. This protection results from the incorporation of the bile acids into mixed micelles with phospholipids and cholesterol. In the mdr2 knock out mouse – the human analog of which is the MDR3 defect reported for a subtype of progressive familial intrahepatic cholestasis[14,15] – phospholipid secretion is defective and phospholipids in bile are practically absent[13]. As a consequence, the biliary epithelium lacks protection by phospholipids against the detergent effects of the bile acids (Figure 2). A form of non-suppurative destructive cholangitis develops which leads to chronic cholestatic liver disease. The liver histopathology is that of a vanishing bile duct lesion. Nieuwkerk *et al.*[13] have used a histological score to study the influence of different bile acids on the progression of this disease. The degree of cholestatic liver disease, evaluated by the histological score, became more severe with time under a control diet without bile acids. Feeding of cholic acid resulted in an even more pronounced histological progression of the disease. In contrast, ursodeoxycholic acid inhibited the histological progression of this cholestatic liver disease (Figure 3).

These studies suggest that ursodeoxycholic acid feeding renders the biliary bile acid composition less detergent and thus diminishes the injurious effects of endogenous bile acids toward bile ducts. In addition to reducing the detergency of the bile acid pool, ursodeoxycholic acid may exert a direct protective effect on cellular membranes. Using electron spin-resonance spectroscopy, Güldütuna *et al.*[16] found that ursodeoxycholic acid protected liver cell plasma membranes against the injurious effects of chenodeoxycholic acid. It was even suggested that tauroursodeoxycholic acid molecules compete for insertion into the membrane with the more hydrophobic bile acids.

A beneficial effect of ursodeoxycholic acid has also been observed in a subgroup of children with progressive familial intrahepatic cholestasis (PFIC) in whom a defect of the MDR3 P-glycoprotein gene is suspected[17].

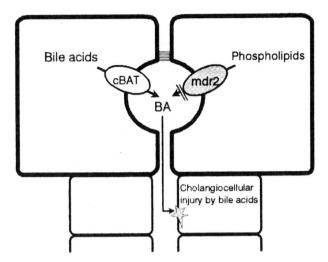

Figure 2 Normal bile acid secretion and defective biliary phospholipid secretion in mice with a disrupted mdr2 P-glycoprotein gene (mdr2 knock out mice; mdr2(−/−)). The biliary epithelium lacks protection by phospholipids against the detergent effects of bile acids (BA). As a consequence, cholangiocellular injury by bile acids and a form of non-suppurative destructive cholangitis develop. cBAT: canalicular bile acid transporter

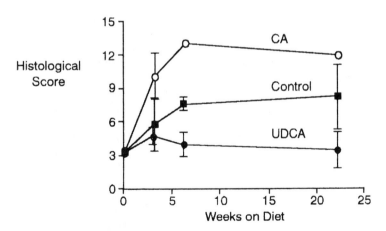

Figure 3 The cholestatic liver injury in mdr2(−/−) mice, evaluated by histological score, progresses under a diet without bile acids (control). Under a diet supplemented with 0.1% cholic acid (CA), the cholestatic liver injury is more pronounced. In contrast, a diet supplemented with 0.5% ursodeoxycholic acid (UDCA) inhibits the progression of the disease. Mean histological scores ± range of values after weaning and after 3, 6 and 22 weeks on the diet. From van Nieuwkerk et al.[13]

STIMULATION OF BILIARY SECRETION

Another important mechanism of action of ursodeoxycholic acid appears to be the stimulation of biliary secretion of hydrophobic bile acids and other potentially toxic cholephils. For an understanding of these effects, the experiments of Kitani et al.[18,19] are of relevance. When the hydrophobic bile acid, taurochenodeoxycholic acid, was infused in the bile fistula rat at a high infusion rate, bile flow decreased and cholestasis occurred. At the same time, LDH excretion into the bile, a sign of toxic liver cell injury, increased. During simultaneous infusion of taurourso- with taurochenodeoxycholic acid, secretion of bile acids and bile flow increased and LDH excretion into the bile was negligible. It may be concluded from these experiments that, in the presence of ursodeoxycholic acid, the liver can secrete a hydrophobic bile acid, such as chenodeoxycholic acid, at a rate that would otherwise be toxic. Thus, ursodeoxycholic acid can overcome the cholestasis caused by hydrophobic bile acids. In isolated hepatocytes, Ohiwa et al.[20] could demonstrate that ursodeoxycholic acid lowers the taurochenodeoxycholic acid content of hepatocytes preloaded with taurochenodeoxycholic acid to a greater extent than taurocholic acid. It also prevented the liberation of LDH from the hepatocytes.

Using the radioactive-labeled bile acid, ^{75}Se homocholic acid taurine, Jazrawi et al.[21] have shown that ursodeoxycholic acid, in patients with primary biliary cirrhosis or primary sclerosing cholangitis, increases the net hepatic excretion rate of this bile acid. This effect of ursodeoxycholic acid on bile acid secretion has recently been measured directly. By duodenal perfusion studies, Stiehl et al.[22] could demonstrate that ursodeoxycholic acid in patients with primary sclerosing cholangitis and elevated bilirubin increases the hourly secretion rate of endogenous bile acids. Most interestingly, phospholipid secretion also increased in these patients. This may be of importance in view of the role of phospholipids in protecting the biliary epithelium against the detergent effects of the bile acids.

The increased biliary secretion of bile acids under ursodeoxycholic acid treatment enhances the elimination of endogenous hydrophobic bile acids from the blood. In a large randomized study together with the group of Poupon[23], we were able to demonstrate that ursodeoxycholic acid treatment decreased chenodeoxycholic acid in the serum of patients with primary biliary cirrhosis while placebo had no effect (Figure 4).

The stimulation of biliary secretion by ursodeoxycholic acid affects not only the secretion of bile acids but also that of other cholephils which are transported by other carrier proteins, for example the multidrug resistance-associated protein 2 (MRP2). Colombo et al.[24] demonstrated that, in patients with cystic fibrosis, the half-time of the hepatic washout of the biliary scintigraphic agent ^{99m}Tc-labeled trimethylbromo-iminodiacetic acid (TMBIDA) decreased after treatment with ursodeoxycholic acid.

The molecular mechanisms by which ursodeoxycholic acid stimulates biliary secretion have not yet been resolved. Beuers et al.[25-27] have shown that tauroursodeoxycholic acid increases cytosolic Ca^{2+}, translocates α-protein kinase C to the membrane, activates α-protein kinase C and, via

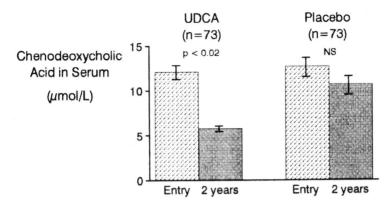

Figure 4 Chenodeoxycholic acid in serum of patients with primary biliary cirrhosis, randomized to ursodeoxycholic acid (UDCA; 13–15 mg/kg^{-1} d^{-1}) or to placebo, at entry and after two years of treatment. Means ± SE. From Poupon *et al.*[23]

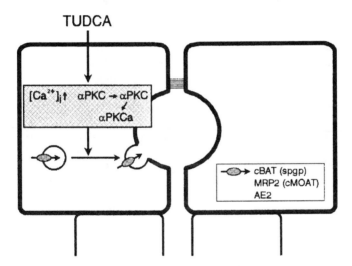

Figure 5 Hypothetical model of the effects of tauroursodeoxycholic acid (TUDCA) on cytosolic free calcium, [Ca^{2+}], α-proteinkinase C (αPKC) and vesicular exocytosis by which carrier proteins (cBAT: canalicular bile acid transporter = spgp: sister of P-glycoprotein; MRP2: multidrug resistance-associated protein 2 = cMOAT: canalicular multispecific organic anion transporter; AE2: chloride–bicarbonate anion exchanger 2) are inserted into the canalicular membrane of the hepatocyte.

these signaling pathways, stimulates hepatocellular exocytosis, a mechanism that is defective in cholestasis (Figure 5). It is tempting to speculate that, via this mechanism, more canalicular carrier proteins, such as the canalicular bile acid transporter (cBAT), the multidrug resistance-associated protein 2 (MRP2) and the chloride–bicarbonate anion exchanger 2 (AE2), could be directed towards and inserted into the canalicular membrane. This would increase the capacity of the hepatocyte for secretion of both bile acids and other organic anions. Schliess et al.[28] have recently identified a signaling pathway, involving the activation of the MAP kinases, Erk-1 and Erk-2, by which ursodeoxycholic acid could stimulate the exocytotic insertion of carrier proteins into the canalicular membrane.

The concept that ursodeoxycholic acid stimulates the insertion of carrier proteins into the canalicular membrane is supported by the findings of Medina et al.[29]. These authors demonstrated that the expression of the chloride–bicarbonate anion exchanger 2 (AE2), which is important for bile-acid-independent bile secretion, is decreased in the liver of patients with primary biliary cirrhosis. Immunostaining of normal liver showed expression of AE2 on bile canaliculi and on the luminal surface of cholangioles and interlobular bile ducts. In patients with primary biliary cirrhosis, AE2 expression was markedly diminished. An immunoreactivity index employed for quantification of AE2 expression was markedly decreased in liver biopsies of untreated patients with primary biliary cirrhosis. In patients with primary biliary cirrhosis on ursodeoxycholic acid treatment, the AE2 immunoreactivity index was significantly improved. Thus, it can be speculated that ursodeoxycholic acid enhances the insertion of the chloride–bicarbonate anion exchanger 2 into the canalicular membrane of hepatocytes and into the apical membrane of cholangiocytes.

It has recently been suggested that ursodeoxycholic acid might also stimulate cholangiocellular bile secretion. There is evidence for uptake both of unconjugated ursodeoxycholic acid[30] and of conjugated bile acids[31] by cholangiocytes. Ursodeoxycholic acid stimulates Ca^{2+}-dependent Cl^- currents in a biliary cell line[32]. If these findings are relevant to native bile duct epithelial cells, ursodeoxycholic acid could, by increasing Cl^- efflux from the apical membrane of bile duct epithelial cells, stimulate cholangiocellular bile formation[33]. Thereby, it could, by diluting hepatocellular bile, diminish cytotoxic effects of hydrophobic bile acids towards the bile duct epithelium.

REDUCTION OF MHC EXPRESSION

Reduction of the expression of major histocompatibility (MHC) antigens on hepatocytes has also been suggested to contribute to the beneficial effects of ursodeoxycholic acid in primary biliary cirrhosis. In primary biliary cirrhosis, MHC class I antigens are aberrantly expressed on hepatocytes and overexpressed on biliary epithelial cells, whereas MHC class II antigens are aberrantly expressed on biliary epithelial cells. Calmus et al.[34] showed that aberrant MHC class I antigen expression on hepatocytes is considerably reduced in patients treated with ursodeoxycholic acid, while there is no detectable change in MHC class II antigens. MHC class I antigens are not only overexpressed on hepatocytes of patients with primary biliary cirrhosis, but also on hepatocytes of patients with extrahepatic cholestasis[35]. Therefore, the effects of ursodeoxycholic acid on MHC expression in the liver of patients with primary biliary cirrhosis could be related to the improvement of cholestasis rather than to a direct effect of ursodeoxycholic acid on the immune system. Whatever the mechanism may be, the decrease of MHC expression may diminish immunologic attack by cytotoxic T cells. The extent to which the effects of ursodeoxycholic acid on MHC expression are relevant to the beneficial therapeutic effects of ursodeoxycholic acid, is still unclear[36].

References

1. Leuschner U, Fischer H, Kurtz W, et al. Ursodeoxycholic acid in primary biliary cirrhosis: results of a controlled double-blind trial. Gastroenterology 1989;97:1268–74.
2. Poupon RE, Balkau B, Eschwege E, Poupon R. A multicenter, controlled trial of ursodiol for the treatment of primary biliary cirrhosis. N Engl J Med 1991;324:1548–54.
3. Heathcote EJ, Cauch-Dudek K, Walker V, et al. The Canadian multicenter double-blind randomized controlled trial of ursodeoxycholic acid in primary biliary cirrhosis. Hepatology 1994;19:1149–56.
4. Lindor KD, Dickson ER, Baldus WP, et al. Ursodeoxycholic acid in the treatment of primary biliary cirrhosis. Gastroenterology 1994;106:1284–90.
5. Combes B, Carithers RL, Maddrey WC, et al. A randomized, double-blind placebo controlled trial of ursodeoxycholic acid in primary biliary cirrhosis. Hepatology 1995;22:759–66.
6. Lindor KD, Therneau TM, Jorgensen RA, Malinchoc M, Dickson ER. Effects of ursodeoxycholic acid on survival in patients with primary biliary cirrhosis. Gastroenterology 1996;110:1515–18.
7. Poupon RE, Lindor KD, Cauch-Dudek K, Dickson ER, Poupon R, Heathcote EJ. Combined analysis of randomized controlled trials of ursodeoxycholic acid in primary biliary cirrhosis. Gastroenterology 1997;113:884–90.
8. Heuman DM. Quantitative estimation of the hydrophobic–hydrophilic balance of mixed bile salt solutions. J Lipid Res 1989;30:719–30.
9. Crosignani A, Podda M, Battezzati PM, et al. Changes in bile acid composition in patients with primary biliary cirrhosis induced by ursodeoxycholic acid administration. Hepatology 1991;14:1000–7.
10. Heuman DM, Bajaj RS. Ursodeoxycholic conjugates protect against disruption of cholesterol-rich membranes by bile salts: a possible physicochemical basis for the hepatoprotective action of ursodeoxycholate. Gastroenterology 1994;106:1333–41.
11. Heuman DM. Disruptive and protective interactions of bile salts, cholesterol:lecithin vesicles, and canalicular membranes. In: Hofmann AF, Paumgartner G, Stiehl A, eds. Bile Acids in Gastroenterology. Lancaster, UK: Kluwer; 1995:283–9.
12. Puglielli L, Amigo L, Arrese M, et al. Protective role of biliary cholesterol and phospholipid lamellae against bile acid-induced cell damage. Gastroenterology 1994;107:244–54.
13. van Nieuwkerk CMJ, Oude Elferink RPJ, Groen AK, et al. Effects of ursodeoxycholate and cholate feeding on liver disease in FVB mice with a disrupted mdr2 P-glycoprotein gene. Gastroenterology 1996;111:165–71.
14. Deleuze JF, Jacquemin E, Dubuisson C, et al. Defect of multidrug-resistance 3 gene expression in a subtype of progressive familial intrahepatic cholestasis. Hepatology 1996;23:904–8.
15. Jacquemin E, de Vree JML, Sturm E, et al. Mutations in the MDR3 gene are responsible for a subtype of progressive familial intrahepatic cholestasis (PFIC). Hepatology 1997;26:248A.
16. Güldütuna S, Zimmer G, Imhof M, Bhatti S, You T, Leuschner U. Molecular aspects of membrane stabilization by ursodeoxycholate. Gastroenterology 1993;104:1736–44.
17. Jacquemin E, Hermans D, Myara A, et al. Ursodeoxycholic acid therapy in pediatric patients with progressive familial intrahepatic cholestasis. Hepatology 1997;25:519–23.
18. Kitani K, Ohta M, Kanai S. Tauroursodeoxycholate prevents the hepatocellular damage caused by other bile salts in the rat. Am J Physiol 1985;248:G407–17.
19. Kitani K. Hepatoprotective effect of ursodeoxycholate in experimental animals. In: Paumgartner G, Stiehl A, Barbara L, Roda E, eds. Strategies for the Treatment of Hepatobiliary Diseases. Dordrecht: Kluwer; 1990:43–56.
20. Ohiwa T, Katagiri K, Hoshino M, Hayakawa T, Nakai T. Tauroursodeoxycholate and tauro-β-muricholate exert cytoprotection by reducing intrahepatocyte taurochenodeoxycholate content. Hepatology 1993;17:470–6.
21. Jazrawi RP, de Caestecker JS, Goggin PM, et al. Kinetics of hepatic bile acid handling in cholestatic liver disease: effect of ursodeoxycholic acid. Gastroenterology 1994;106:134–42.

22. Stiehl A, Rudolph G, Sauer P, Theilmann L. Biliary secretion of bile acids and lipids in primary sclerosing cholangitis. Influence of cholestasis and effect of ursodeoxycholic acid treatment. J Hepatol 1995;23:283–9.
23. Poupon RE, Chrétien Y, Poupon R, Paumgartner G. Serum bile acids in primary biliary cirrhosis: effect of ursodeoxycholic acid therapy. Hepatology 1993;17:599–604.
24. Colombo C, Castellani MR, Balistreri WF, Seregni E, Assaido ML, Giunta A. Scintigraphic documentation of an improvement in hepatobiliary excretory function after treatment with ursodeoxycholic acid in patients with cystic fibrosis and associated liver disease. Hepatology 1992;15:677–84.
25. Beuers U, Nathanson MH, Boyer JL. Effects of tauroursodeoxycholic acid on cytosolic Ca^{++} signals in isolated rat hepatocytes. Gastroenterology 1993;104:604–12.
26. Beuers U, Nathanson MH, Isales CM, Boyer JL. Tauroursodeoxycholic acid stimulates hepatocellular exocytosis and mobilizes extracellular Ca^{++}, mechanisms defective in cholestasis. J Clin Invest 1993;92:2984–93.
27. Beuers U, Throckmorton DC, Anderson MS, et al. Tauroursodeoxycholic acid activates protein kinase C in isolated rat hepatocytes. Gastroenterology 1996;110:1553–63.
28. Schliess F, Kurz AK, vom Dahl S, Häussinger D. Mitogen-activated protein kinases mediate the stimulation of bile acid secretion by tauroursodeoxycholate in rat liver. Gastroenterology 1997;113:1306–14.
29. Medina JF, Martínez-Anso E, Vázquez JJ, Prieto J. Decreased anion exchanger 2 immunoreactivity in the liver of patients with primary biliary cirrhosis. Hepatology 1997;25:12–17.
30. Lamri Y, Erlinger S, Dumont M, Roda A, Feldmann G. Immunoperoxidase localization of bile salts in rat liver cells. J Clin Invest 1988;82:1173–82.
31. Lazaridis K, Pham L, de Groen P, Dawson P, Larusso NF. Rat cholangiocytes express the ileal Na^+-dependent taurocholate co-transporter. Hepatology 1996;24:897A.
32. Shimokura GH, McGill JM, Schlenker, T, Fitz JG. Ursodeoxycholate increases cytosolic calcium concentration and activates Cl^- currents in a biliary cell line. Gastroenterology 1995;109:965–72.
33. Roman R, Schlenker T, Fitz JG. Ursodeoxycholic acid activates Ca^{2+}-dependent Cl^- currents in a human biliary cell line. In: Paumgartner G, Stiehl A, Gerok W, eds. Bile Acids in Hepatobiliary Diseases: Basic Research and Clinical Application. Dordrecht: Kluwer Academic Publishers; 1997:219–23.
34. Calmus Y, Gane R, Rouger P, Poupon R. Hepatic expression of class I and class II major histocompatibility molecules in primary biliary cirrhosis: effect of ursodeoxycholic acid. Hepatology 1990;11:12–15.
35. Calmus Y, Arvieux C, Gane R, et al. Cholestasis induces major histocompatibility complex class I in hepatocytes. Gastroenterology 1992;102:1371–7.
36. Neuberger J. Immune effects of ursodeoxycholic acid. In: Berg P, Lohse AW, Tiegs G, Wendel A, eds. Autoimmune Liver Disease. Dordrecht: Kluwer Academic Publishers; 1997:93–103.

18
Ursodiol and combination therapy

R. L. CARITHERS JR.

INTRODUCTION

A variety of therapeutic agents have been proposed for treatment of patients with primary biliary cirrhosis (PBC). However, when carefully studied in controlled clinical trails, most have been found to be ineffective or too toxic for widespread use. In contrast, ursodiol therapy is remarkably well tolerated and provides dramatic improvement in the biochemical features of PBC. Nevertheless, questions remain about the overall efficacy of the drug in improving patients' symptoms, arresting histological progression of the disease, and, most importantly, improving survival and delaying the need for liver transplantation. Ursodiol also has been combined with a variety of other agents, including corticosteriods, colchicine, and methotrexate, in an attempt to enhance favorable effects on the outcome of patients with PBC.

The purpose of this review is to critically evaluate the controlled clinical trials in which ursodiol, alone or in combination with other agents, has been studied in patients with PBC. Most of these trials have compared ursodiol therapy with placebo therapy. However, a few studies have systematically compared ursodiol alone with combination therapy using ursodiol and another potential therapeutic agent.

URSODIOL ALONE

The potential benefit of ursodiol was suggested by the observation that liver function tests improved in patients with chronic active hepatitis who were being treated with ursodiol for concomitant gallstones. Small pilot studies confirmed these observations and provided the basis for large multicenter trials designed to critically examine the role of ursodiol therapy in patients with primary biliary cirrhosis. Although numerous placebo-controlled randomized trials of ursodiol have been performed, 4 large studies provide the bulk of our data on the efficacy of ursodiol in PBC. Throughout this discussion, they will be referred to as the French trial[1], the Canadian trial[2], the Mayo Clinic trial[3], and, the US multicenter study[4].

Table 1 Exclusion criteria for the four multi-center trials

	French	Canadian	Mayo Clinic	United States
Serum bilirubin (mg/dl)	> 8.9		*	> 20
Serum albumin (g/dl)	< 2.5		*	
Variceal bleeding	X		X	X
Diuretic resistant ascites			X	X
Encephalopathy			X	X

* Patients were not excluded for specific levels of bilirubin or albumin but were not entered if the need for liver transplantation was anticipated within 1 year based on predicted survival determined by the Mayo Clinic prognostic model.

Table 2 Baseline values in the four multicenter trials

	French	Canadian	Mayo Clinic	United States
Number	146	222	180	151
Age*	56 ± 1	56 ± 12	53 ± 9	49 ± 10
Women (%)	92	93	89	89
Serum bilirubin (mg/dl)	1.3 ± 0.02	2.1 ± 3.0	1.9 ± 2.3	2.1 ± 2.8
Mayo risk score	4.9 ± 0.01	4.6 ± 1.3	5.2 ± 1.1	4.7 ± 1.2
Histological stage (%)				
I and II	53	45	32	33
III and IV	47	55	68	67
Daily ursodiol dose (mg)	13–15	14	13–15	10–12
Administration (per day)	2	1	4	1

* Unless otherwise indicated, values reflect mean ± standard deviation.

Study design

The patients included in these trials all had classical clinical, biochemical, and histological features of PBC. All studies required that patients have elevated alkaline phosphatase values prior to study entry[a]. In addition, each of the trials required that patients have a positive antimitochondrial antibody test[b].

Patients were excluded from each of the trials if they had evidence of another type of liver disease or if they had recently been taking other potential therapeutic agents, such as colchicine. Three of the trials excluded patients with far-advanced liver disease whereas no attempt was made to do so in the Canadian multicenter trial. See Table 1.

Despite these varying exclusion criteria, the patients in each of the four trials were quite similar at study entry (Table 2). Women accounted for the

[a] For inclusion in the Canadian multicenter trial, the alkaline phosphatase values had to be above the upper limit of normal for the local hospital laboratory. The Mayo Clinic study and US multicenter trial required alkaline phosphatase values 1.5 times the upper limit of normal and the French multicenter trial required alkaline phosphatase values more than 2 times the upper limit of normal.
[b] The US multicenter trial allowed entry of patients with classical features of PBC who had a negative antimitochondrial antibody if they had convincing evidence to exclude extrahepatic biliary obstruction. The seven patients in this category had identical clinical features and outcome compared with the 144 AMA-positive patients.

vast majority of patients in each of the trials. The French and Canadian patients were older, particularly when compared with patients in the US multicenter trial. The French patients were more homogeneous and had milder clinical and histological manifestations of disease than patients entered into the other three trials. However, somewhat paradoxically, they had higher Mayo scores than patients entered into the Canadian and US multicenter trials, who had higher mean bilirubin values at study entry[c].

Patients in the French, Canadian, and Mayo Clinic trials received Urso® whereas patients in the US multicenter trial received Actigall®. The administration of drugs ranged from 4 times daily in the Mayo Clinic study to once daily at bedtime in the Canadian and US multicenter trials. Although patients in the US multicenter trial were prescribed 10–12 mg of ursodiol in a single daily dose at bedtime, ursodeoxycholic acid enrichment of the bile acid pool was identical to that seen in the Mayo Clinic trial in which patients received 13–15 mg ursodiol daily in 4 divided doses[d].

In the French, Canadian, and US multicenter trials, patients received ursodiol or placebo for 2 years. At the end of 2 years, patients were offered open-label ursodiol and were then followed for an additional 2–3 years. In the Mayo trial, 180 patients were recruited over a four-year period from April 1988 until June 1992. After the 132nd randomized patient had received 2 years of follow-up on the initial study drug, all patients were offered open-label ursodiol for an additional 2–3 years. Thus, many patients remained on placebo for up to 4 years whereas a minority received placebo for less than 2 years.

In summary, these independent multicenter trials recruited patients with remarkably similar prognostic features. Based on the Mayo Clinic prognostic model for PBC, the anticipated survival of patients was virtually identical at 2 years, with slightly worse expected survival over time among patients entered in the Mayo Clinic trial.

Results

Each of these 4 two-year trials was designed to evaluate the efficacy of ursodiol therapy in alleviating symptoms, improving biochemical measures of disease activity, and reducing histological progression of disease. None was designed to determine the impact of ursodiol therapy on patient survival. However, since survival is such an important issue in clinical trials, each of these studies was critically reassessed to evaluate the impact of ursodiol therapy on symptoms, biochemistry, histology, and survival.

---

[c] This may in part have been due to very high bilirubin values in a few patients which skewed the mean entry values higher. In the Canadian trial, the median bilirubin value at entry was 1.1 mg/dl compared with a mean value of 2.1 mg/dl. Median and mean entry bilirubin values were 1.0 and 2.1 mg/dl, respectively, in the US multicenter trial. These patients also were younger than patients in the other three trials.

[d] Duodenal bile was collected only from patients in the Mayo and US multicenter trials. Samples from both centers were assayed under code in a single laboratory (Alan Hofmann). The mean UDCA level at 2 years was 40% in the Mayo patients compared with 39% among patients in the US multicenter trial.

Symptoms

The two symptoms directly addressed by the trials were fatigue and pruritus. In three of the studies, numerical grading systems were used to compare the degree of fatigue and pruritus at various time points. In none of the trials was ursodiol therapy associated with improvement in patients' perception of fatigue. Similarly, when the percentages of patients experiencing pruritus and pruritus scores were evaluated, therapeutic benefit from ursodiol therapy was seen in only one trial[1]. However, when patients' diaries were assessed for the amount of cholestyramine required for symptom relief, and the number of patients who developed disabling pruritus were included, ursodiol appeared to have a clear impact on pruritus in both the Canadian and US multicenter trials[4,5]. Thus, the Mayo Clinic study was the only trial in which some benefit of ursodiol therapy on pruritus could not be demonstrated.

Biochemistry

Ursodiol therapy was associated with dramatic improvement in biochemical measures of disease activity. This was most prominent in measures of cholestasis such as alkaline phosphatase and γ-glutamyl transpeptidase levels. However, there were also significant improvements in AST and ALT values and total serum bilirubin levels. Serum cholesterol and IgM values also showed significant improvement in ursodiol recipients in two trials[1,2]. However, in the two-year duration of these trials, there was no improvement in serum albumin or prothrombin time values.

Histology

The degree of histological stage was categorized in three of the trials using the Ludwig criteria[6] whereas, in the Canadian trial, the biopsies were staged on the basis of fibrosis alone (stage I, no fibrosis; stage II, periportal fibrosis; stage III, fibrosis with septae; and stage IV, cirrhosis)[2]. In the French trial, 95 pre- and post-treatment biopsies were compared. Various measures of inflammation, cholestasis, and ductular changes improved or failed to worsen more often in ursodiol-treated patients compared with placebo recipients. However, there was no significant change in the degree of fibrosis. Nevertheless, more ursodiol recipients showed histological improvement and fewer worsened during the trial compared with placebo recipients[1]. In the Canadian trial, both ductular proliferation and paucity appeared to be favorably influenced by ursodiol therapy but there was no effect on fibrosis or histological staging[2]. A total of 122 paired biopsies were available for comparison in the US multicenter trial. In this trial, favorable histological changes were primarily limited to patients who had serum bilirubin values less than 2 mg/dl at study entry. In the 86 paired biopsies in these patients, ursodiol therapy was associated with improved measures of inflammation and average score in those with stage I and II disease at study entry. However, in patients with stage III or IV disease at study entry, there was a significant improvement in fibrosis among ursodiol recipients. Although fewer ursodiol-treated patients in the entire trial had histological progression during the study, this was not statistically significant[4]. Finally, in the Mayo

Clinic trial, improvement in neither inflammation nor histological stage was seen in ursodiol-treated patients compared with placebo recipients[7]. In summary, ursodiol therapy is accompanied by some improvement in inflammation and ductular changes; however, fibrosis and histological stage do not appear to be favorably influenced by two years of therapy.

Survival

None of these clinical trials was specifically designed to assess the influence of ursodiol therapy on patient mortality. In fact, by the end of the 2 year phases of these trials, only 32 of the evaluable 553 patients randomized had died prior to transplantation (5.8%)[f]. Although there were more deaths in the placebo group, the numbers of hepatic deaths were the same in patients randomized to ursodiol compared with those who received placebo. Because of the low mortality, the relatively small number of patients in each of these trials, and the short duration of follow-up, these results are not unexpected. In fact, if ursodiol therapy prevented 50% of the deaths with mortality rates this low, a total of 2582 patients would be required to demonstrate such a difference in a clinical trial[g].

At the end of the two-year randomized trials, each of the groups offered patients open-label ursodiol and continued follow-up for an additional 2–3 years[h]. This extended the duration of follow-up to 4–5 years for the French, Canadian, and US studies and to 5–7 years for some patients in the Mayo Clinic trial. Poupon and colleagues reported a significant reduction in deaths and referral for liver transplantation among patients who remained on continuous ursodiol therapy for 4 years compared with those who received placebo for 2 years followed by ursodiol for 2 years[8]. However, the difference consisted primarily of patients referred for transplantation. There were 4 pretransplant deaths (3 of hepatic origin) among those on continuous ursodiol compared with 7 deaths (5 of hepatic origin) in patients originally randomized to placebo. In contrast, there were only 4 liver transplants (or referrals) in those on continuous ursodiol vs. 13 transplants (or referrals) among those originally assigned to placebo. The patients who originally received placebo had significantly higher serum bilirubin values at the end of the two-year randomized trial than those who received continuous ursodiol. One wonders if physicians referring patients for transplantation may have been biased by these elevated bilirubin values and thus confounded the results. In contrast to the results from this extended trial, there was no difference in time to transplantation or death among patients followed longer in the Canadian or US multicenter trials[9,10]. Finally, there was a trend toward increased transplant-free survival among continuous ursodiol recipients in the extended follow-up of patients entered into the Mayo Clinic trial[11]. Furthermore, in both the Mayo Clinic and US multicenter trials, the actual survival of patients was superior to that predicted by their Mayo

---

[f] Deaths were not reported in the French trial.

[g] Sample size calculated assuming 5% mortality predicted at 2 years by the Mayo model, $p < 0.05$, and power of 0.9.

[h] Only the first 100 patients randomized in the Canadian trial were offered open-label ursodiol.

scores at study entry, as indirect evidence for a favorable effect of ursodiol on patients' survival[11,12].

Based on the Mayo scores of patients entered into these 4 trials, 15% of patients would be predicted to die within 4 years and 20% within 5 years after study entry. Assuming that ursodiol prevented half of these deaths, a total of 696 patients would be required to demonstrate such an effect on patient mortality. Thus, although none of the individual trials were of sufficient size to demonstrate an effect of ursodiol therapy on patient survival, the potential for a combined analysis of data from the various trials became evident.

This combined analysis revealed a significant increase in transplant-free survival among those patients who remained on continuous ursodiol therapy compared with patients who originally received placebo followed by ursodiol therapy[13]. This was most apparent among patients with serum bilirubin values above 1.4 mg/dl at study entry and in those with cirrhosis. Within 4 years there were 22 liver transplants and 25 deaths among those originally randomized to ursodiol compared with 32 transplants and 34 deaths among those assigned to placebo. Although the potential confounding of liver transplantation on patient survival can never be entirely resolved, these are the best data we will ever have regarding the effect of ursodiol therapy on patient survival.

COMBINATION THERAPY

A number of trials have been initiated to examine the possibility that combining ursodiol with other agents might be even more beneficial to patients with primary biliary cirrhosis. The combinations studied to date in controlled clinical trials include ursodiol–colchicine, ursodiol–prednisolone, and ursodiol–methotrexate.

Ursodiol–colchicine

Two randomized trials of ursodiol–colchicine compared with ursodiol alone have been published. In both studies, patients were initially treated with ursodiol. In one trial, after 30 months of daily 600 mg ursodiol therapy, 22 patients were randomly allocated to continue ursodiol alone or to receive ursodiol plus 1 mg colchicine daily for 2 years[14]. In another larger trial, 74 patients with PBC who had been treated for at least 8 months with ursodiol but continued to have abnormal LFTs were randomly allocated to continue on ursodiol and a placebo or receive ursodiol plus 1 mg colchicine daily for 2 years[15]. In the latter trial, endoscopy and liver biopsies were performed at study entry and at the conclusion of the 2-year treatment course. In the smaller Japanese trial, all liver function tests showed significant improvement in patients on the combination therapy compared with those on ursodiol alone[14]. In contrast, in the larger French trial, there were no differences in symptoms, biochemical features, or histological features except lobular inflammation between the two treatment groups[15]. However, patients who received the combination therapy demonstrated a trend toward reduced progression of esophageal varices during the trial.

Ursodiol–prednisolone

A 9-month course of ursodiol therapy was compared with ursodiol plus 10 mg of prednisolone daily in one small randomized trial of 30 patients[16]. The authors reported dramatic improvement in the histological features of PBC on follow-up biopsies in patients on combination therapy. However, these changes were limited to periportal and lobular inflammation and piecemeal necrosis. Bile ductular changes and fibrosis were not affected.

Ursodiol–methotrexate

The outcome of patients treated with ursodiol–methotrexate was compared with that of patients in the previous ursodiol trial in a small pilot study of 32 patients at the Mayo Clinic[17]. The combination therapy was not associated with any demonstrable improvement in symptoms, laboratory studies, or histological features compared with the historical controls. During the study, 7 patients had to discontinue the combination therapy because of intolerable side-effects. These included mouth ulcers, extreme fatigue, and hair loss in one patient each. However, the most common side-effect was pulmonary toxicity, which occurred in 4 patients and resulted in hospitalization in 2.

A total of 160 patients have been enrolled in the US multicenter trial of ursodiol–methotrexate versus ursodiol–placebo. In this study, patients with well-characterized primary biliary cirrhosis who have serum bilirubin values < 3 mg/dl are treated for 6 months with 13–15 mg/kg ursodiol and then randomized to receive combination therapy versus ursodiol–placebo for at least 5 years. Patients have now been followed for 1–48 months. Long-term follow-up of 7–9 years is planned. To date, no pulmonary toxicity has been seen in this large trial despite the fact that patients are being followed prospectively with pulmonary diffusing capacity studies.

SUMMARY

Ursodeoxycholic acid appears to an effective and remarkably safe treatment for patients with primary biliary cirrhosis. Patients at all stages of disease appear to benefit from ursodiol therapy. Some studies suggest that biochemical and histological improvement is most apparent in patients with milder disease[4]. However, patients with more advanced disease, especially those with elevated bilirubin values and cirrhosis on biopsy, are most immediately affected with improvement in survival or delay in the need for liver transplantation[12]. Combined therapy of ursodiol with other agents, such as colchicine and methotrexate, shows promise of additional benefits to patients with primary biliary cirrhosis. However, these treatments should be limited to carefully controlled clinical trials until the benefits and toxicity are well defined.

References

1. Poupon RE, Balkau B, Eschwege E, *et al.* A multicenter, controlled trial of ursodiol for the treatment of primary biliary cirrhosis. N Engl J Med 1991;324:1548–54.

2. Heathcote EJ, Cauch-Dudek K, Walker V, *et al.* The Canadian multicenter double-blind randomized controlled trial of ursodeoxycholic acid in primary biliary cirrhosis. Hepatology 1994;19:1149–56.
3. Lindor KD, Dickson ER, Baldus WP, *et al.* Ursodeoxycholic acid in the treatment of primary biliary cirrhosis. Gastroenterology 1994;106:1284–90.
4. Combes B, Carithers RL Jr, Maddrey WC, *et al.* A randomized, double-blind, placebo-controlled trial of ursodeoxycholic acid in primary biliary cirrhosis. Hepatology 1995;22:759–66.
5. Ghant CN, Cauch-Dudek K, Heathcote EJ, and the Canadian PBC trial group. Ursodeoxycholic acid therapy and fatigue in primary biliary cirrhosis. Hepatology 1997;26:438A (Abstract).
6. Ludwig J, Dickson ER, McDonald GSA. Staging of chronic nonsuppurative destructive cholangitis (syndrome of primary biliary cirrhosis). Virchows Arch Pathol Anat 1978;379:103–12.
7. Batts KP, Jorgensen RA, Dickson ER, Lindor KD. Effects of ursodeoxycholic acid on hepatic inflammation and histological stage in patients with primary biliary cirrhosis. Am J Gastroenterol 1996;91:2314–17.
8. Poupon RE, Poupon R, Balkau B, *et al.* Ursodiol for the long-term treatment of primary biliary cirrhosis. N Engl J Med 1994;330:1342–7.
9. Kilmurry MR, Heathcote EJ, Cauch-Dudek K, *et al.* Is the Mayo model for predicting survival useful after the introduction of ursodeoxycholic acid treatment for primary biliary cirrhosis? Hepatology 1996;23:1148–53.
10. Carithers RL Jr, Luketic VA, Peters M, *et al.* Extended follow-up of patients in the U.S. multicenter trial of ursodeoxycholic acid for primary biliary cirrhosis. Gastoenterology 1996;110:A1163(Abstract).
11. Lindor KD, Therneau TM, Jorgensen RA, Malinchoc M, Dickson ER. Effects of ursode-oxycholic acid on survival in patients with primary biliary cirrhosis. Gastroenterology 1996;110:1515–18.
12. Emond M, Carithers RL Jr, Luketic VA, *et al.* Does ursodeoxycholic acid improve survival in patients with primary biliary cirrhosis? Comparison of outcome in the U.S. multicenter trial to expected survival using the Mayo Clinic prognostic model. Hepatology 1996;24:168A(Abstract).
13. Poupon RE, Lindor KD, Cauch-Dudek K, Dickson ER, Poupon R, Heathcote EJ. Combined analysis of randomized controlled trials of ursodeoxycholic acid in primary biliary cirrhosis. Gastroenterology 1997;113:884–90.
14. Ikeda T, Tozuka S, Noguchi O, *et al.* Effects of additional administration of colchicine in ursodeoxycholic acid-treated patients with primary biliary cirrhosis: a prospective random-ized study. J Hepatol 1996;24:88–94.
15. Poupon RE, Huet PM, Poupon R, *et al.* A randomized trial comparing colchicine and ursodeoxycholic acid combination to ursodeoxycholic acid in primary biliary cirrhosis. Hepatology 1996;24:1098–103.
16. Leuschner M, Guldutuna S, You T, Hubner K, Bhatti S, Leuschner U. Ursodeoxycholic acid and prednisolone versus ursodeoxycholic acid and placebo in the treatment of early stages of primary biliary cirrhosis. J Hepatol 1996;25:49–57.
17. Lindor KD, Dickson ER, Jorgensen RA, *et al.* The combination of ursodeoxycholic acid and methotrexate for patients with primary biliary cirrhosis: the results of a pilot study. Hepatology 1995;22:1158–62.

19
Primary biliary cirrhosis transplantation and recurrent disease

J. NEUBERGER

INTRODUCTION

Despite the many recent advances in understanding the pathophysiology of primary biliary cirrhosis (PBC) and the developments in therapy, no drug has yet been shown to arrest the relentless progression of the syndrome[1], so many patients will develop end-stage disease. Therefore, PBC remains one of the major indications for liver transplantation[2]. Most centers are reporting 1- and 5-year survival results in excess of 80%. In this chapter, the indications, timing, results and evidence for recurrence of disease in the graft will be discussed.

INDICATIONS

As for other liver diseases, the general indications for liver replacement are either an intolerable and unacceptable quality of life (because of the liver disease) or an anticipated length of life less than one year (again, because of liver disease). In PBC, the two major symptoms which may render the patient's quality of life intolerable are lethargy and pruritus. Although the severity of the lethargy may be severe, this is a rare indication for transplantation. It is important to exclude treatable causes of lethargy, such as co-existing thyroid disease, adrenal insufficiency, and celiac disease, all of which are associated with PBC[2]. Sometimes, the medications, including antihistamines given for the treatment of pruritus, may induce lethargy. As would be anticipated in any patient with a chronic progressive disease, depression is not uncommon, so it is important to distinguish depression which arises as a consequence of the lethargy from depression leading to lethargy which may respond well to appropriate therapy. However, the symptoms of lethargy associated with PBC differ from those associated with depression[3]. Intractable pruritus is another valid indication for grafting but

155

Table 1 Indications for liver transplantation in PBC

Clinical:	Intractable pruritus
	Intractable lethargy
	Recurrent variceal hemorrhage
	Ascites difficult to control medically
	Spontaneous bacterial peritonitis
	Hepatic encephalopathy
	Progressive malnutrition*
	Progressive hepatic osteopenia*
	Significant hepatopulmonary syndrome*
	Development of hepatocellular carcinoma*
Serological:	Serum bilirubin $>170 \, \mu$mol/L
	Serum albumin <25 g/L

* These indications may also be contraindications.

it is essential to ensure that all treatments have been tried; of those patients referred for transplantation to the Birmingham Liver Unit for 'intractable' pruritus, it has been possible to treat the itching medically in over half and so defer the need for grafting.

Those clinical features that suggest the prognosis is limited to less than one year are listed in Table 1. It will be noted that some of the indications are, paradoxically, also contraindications: thus, progressive osteopenia, malnutrition, hepatopulmonary syndrome and development of hepatocellular carcinoma may all, in themselves, be valid indications for transplantation, but extensive hepatocellular carcinoma or advanced hepatopulmonary syndrome may preclude a successful outcome after surgery.

There are few absolute contraindications to transplantation: active infection will usually require treatment before grafting can be successfully undertaken. Few centers will offer transplantation to those who are HIV positive as longer-term survival is low. Patients with PBC are at risk of developing both hepatic and extrahepatic cancers[4]. The finding of a small incidental hepatocellular carcinoma, often by routine screening with serum α-fetoprotein estimations or routine ultrasound, is a clear indication for grafting: where there is extrahepatic spread, multiple nodules (>5), large tumors (>5 cm) or vascular invasion, grafting is contraindicated[5]. With respect to extrahepatic cancers, Penn[6] has published data from the registry on renal allograft recipients: of those with cancers present before transplantation, there were high ($>26\%$) recurrence rates with bladder carcinomas, sarcomas, renal cancers, malignant melanomas and non-melanomatous cancers and sarcomas. A low recurrence rate ($<10\%$) occurred with lymphomas, uterine, cervical and thyroid cancers. Intermediate rates were found with breast cancer and with bowel cancer.

TIMING OF TRANSPLANTATION

Timing of transplantation in PBC is probably easier than in any other indication, since, for most patients, the disease runs a fairly predictable course. Since the initial observation by Schaffner and colleagues[7], serum bilirubin has been recognized as a simple and reliable marker of disease progression. Once the serum bilirubin reaches 150 µmol/L, life expectancy is about 12–18 months. The advent of various prognostic models has allowed for more accurate assessment of patient survival. However, while these models are useful when applied to a population, care must be taken when extrapolating the prognosis derived from an estimated probability of survival to an individual[8]: the confidence intervals are relatively wide. Models cannot take into account other factors which the clinician, consciously or subconsciously, uses, such as the degree of malnutrition, the difficulty in controlling ascites or the presence of encephalopathy.

Although many authors (including this one) have stated that liver transplantation should be done when the anticipated survival is less than one year, there is little objective evidence to defend this time interval. Timing of the procedure must depend on optimizing the benefits and minimizing the risks of major surgery. The prognostic variables and their importance which predict survival *without* transplantation differ from those which predict survival *after* transplantation[9]. Using statistical modeling, we have tried to identify at which point, during the progression of PBC, the probability of survival is greater after transplantation than without grafting; we found that the optimal time to transplant[10] is when the serum bilirubin is about 170 µmol/L.

It is important that models are used as an aid to decision making and not as an alternative to the clinical decision-making progress.

Because of the shortage of donor livers, the patient may have a considerable wait from the time of listing until a suitable organ becomes available, and therefore the time of listing of patients for transplantation must allow for this often-prolonged wait. The duration of waiting for a suitable graft will depend, not only on the country where the transplant will be done, but also on the size of the patient and the recipient's blood group. Our own recent experience has found that, for adult patients listed for transplantation, the on-list mortality was 9%[11]; however, patient characteristics will affect the length of wait on the list so that small patients with blood group O will wait on average 6–8 months whereas a large patient with blood group A will wait a median of 2–3 months. In North America, waiting periods are often considerably longer.

Patients should be referred to a transplant unit in sufficient time for a full and mutual assessment and once the patient and clinician have reached a conclusion, the patient should be listed at a time when the patient will actually be grafted and when not too ill.

ALLOGRAFT REJECTION

Patients grafted for PBC are at greater risk of developing both acute cellular rejection and chronic ductopenic rejection. Thus, in our own series of primary adult liver grafts of patients transplanted between 1994 and 1997, acute early rejection occurred in 43% of patients grafted for PBC, compared with 20% for those grafted for alcoholic liver disease and 12% for hepatitis B-related liver disease[12]. Similarly, Farges et al.[13] reported that acute cellular rejection occurred in 45% of those grafted for PBC compared with 30% for those grafted for alcoholic liver disease or primary liver cell cancer. Whether this observation is of any clinical importance is uncertain since there is no clear evidence that early (before 28 days following transplantation) rejection is associated with a worse outcome, either for the patient or the graft. However, several studies[14,15] have shown that transplantation for PBC is a significant risk factor for the development of chronic ductopenic rejection. Our own studies[16] suggest that patients grafted for PBC have an odds ratio of 10.6 for developing chronic rejection. Since chronic rejection is associated with graft loss, it is possible that immunosuppression should be modified, with perhaps the aim of achieving higher concentrations of cyclosporin or tacrolimus.

It is not clear why patients with PBC are at greater risk of developing allograft rejection. One possibility is that the genetic susceptibility that predisposes the patient to develop PBC may also be the same as that which allows for rejection. Another possibility is that the biliary epithelial cells are the immune targets both in PBC and in rejection so that PBC patients are already sensitized to biliary antigens. The latter option is supported by the observation that primary sclerosing cholangitis (PSC), another disease where the biliary epithelial cells are believed to be the immunological target, is also a risk factor for allograft rejection.

QUALITY OF LIFE AFTER TRANSPLANTATION

After transplantation, the quality of life for the patient usually shows considerable improvement, although it must be stressed that life is never normal. There is usually rapid resolution of the lethargy and of pruritus. Thus, Nevasa and colleagues[17] studied 26 patients grafted for PBC who had survived for more than two years. In their patients, the most commonly reported symptom was bone pain (in 58%) and nearly one third developed bone fractures; this is an alarmingly high rate which compares with less than 1% in our own series. Complications relating to immunosuppression (such as arterial hypertension and renal impairment) occurred in half the patients. The quality of life, as estimated by the Karnovsky index, was good with a median index of 90 (range 60–100). Self-assessed health perception was largely good, with over one third reporting a very good quality of life and only one patient reporting a bad health perception. Findings from the Nottingham Health Profile identified problems mainly in the domains of sleep, emotional reactions and physical mobility.

Thus, while quality of life after transplantation is good, there will be continuing problems which require proper monitoring.

DISEASE RECURRENCE

The diagnosis of PBC in the native liver is made on the basis of clinical, biochemical, immunological and histological findings. However, the conventional diagnostic criteria which define PBC in the native liver may not be applicable to the graft. There are many causes of graft dysfunction which

Table 2 Series reporting recurrence of PBC

Source	No. of PBC patients	No. (%) with recurrence	Comments
Mayo Clinic[31]	60	5 (8%)	Diagnosed 2–6 years post-OLT
Innsbruck[32]	8	2 (25%)	6–12 months post-OLT
Kings College Hospital, London[20]	33	8 (24%)	Patients studied > 5 years post-OLT
Paris[33]	69	6 (9%)	Patients studied > 1 year post-OLT
Pittsburgh[25]	421	54 (13%)	8% at 5 years, 22% at 10 years
Birmingham[23]	81	16 (20%)	Review of protocol annual biopsies
UCSF/OHSU[27]	n/a	5	Study of patients with hepatic granulomas

n/a = not available.

may lead to cholestatic liver function tests and to histological evidence of immune-mediated bile duct damage. Persistence of antimitochondrial antibodies (AMA) does not prove the recurrence of disease: there is no evidence that these antibodies are pathogenic. Furthermore, the expression of putative recurrent disease may be modified by the altered HLA phenotype of the donor liver and by the administration of immunosuppressive drugs. AMA persist after transplantation with a specificity similar to that seen prior to grafting.[18]. Diagnosis of recurrent disease must depend on a combination of clinical, serological and, above all, histological features.

The initial report of recurrent PBC was based on three patients who had developed clinical, serological and histological features of recurrent disease[19]; a follow-up study identified a further three patients[20]. In all instances, the AMA were detectable after transplantation and liver histology showed bile duct damage with a predominantly lymphoid infiltrate around an enlarged irregular portal tract. There was evidence of increased deposition of copper-associated protein in the absence of histological evidence of cholestasis and without biliary obstruction. One patient died 5 years later and examination of the failed allograft showed features of chronic ductopenic rejection and nodular regenerative hyperplasia[21]; the authors concluded that there was no evidence of recurrent PBC, although the features of recurrent disease may have been masked by the process of ductopenic rejection.

Since these initial reports, there have been many reports of recurrent disease in the allograft (Table 2). Not all series have, however, reported recurrent PBC: thus, in our own experience in Birmingham, a small initial study[22] looking at the histological features on protocol annual liver biopsies concluded that there was no evidence of recurrent disease; a later study involving more patients with a longer follow-up reached opposite conclusions[23]. Similarly, an early study from Pittsburgh suggested that there was no evidence in failed allografts that PBC recurred[24]; however, a later study, looking also at protocol biopsies, reported that some patients had recurrent disease[25]. Other groups have had a similar experience. The only major large-scale study evaluating protocol biopsies that has failed to find evidence of recurrent PBC is from the Netherlands[26]. The histological findings of 19 patients grafted for PBC were compared with 14 patients grafted for other

159

indications; while about one third of patients in each group had evidence of bile-duct damage, in none was there evidence of recurrent disease. Granulomas were present in some but these were not a feature of recurrent disease. In contrast, a study from San Francisco[27] showed that while there were many causes for liver granulomas in the allograft, recurrent PBC was the explanation in 12% of cases with hepatic granulomas; the majority of granulomas were parenchymal, unlike those associated with recurrent PBC which were located in the portal areas.

There is no clear explanation for the discrepancy in these findings: one possibility is that the disease recurs in only a small proportion of patients and the histological lesions may be patchy so smaller studies may miss features of recurrent disease. Another possibility is that the immunosuppressive protocol may affect the pattern of disease recurrence: we found that patients receiving tacrolimus-based immunosuppression were more likely to develop recurrence earlier and more aggressively than those receiving cyclosporin-based treatment[28]. In contrast, Yoshida and colleagues suggested that features of recurrent disease became apparent only when cyclosporin levels fell below the target range[29]. Similarly, Mazariegos et al.[30] reported that, during a prospective study of withdrawal of immunosuppression, two patients had to discontinue the study beause of the development of recurrent PBC. It is of interest that the Dutch group tends to use triple therapy whereas we ourselves and the Kings College Hospital group use less-aggressive immunosuppression. Clearly, further work is required to resolve these issues.

Whether recurrent disease is of clinical importance is less clear. A recent analysis from Pittsburgh[25] suggested that histological features were found in 1.1% at 1 year, 7.9% at 5 years and 21.6% at 10 years. Although the median follow-up was 91 months from the time of transplantation and 16 months from the time of diagnosis of recurrent disease, the group found no evidence that disease recurrence had a significant impact on either patient or graft survival. We have been treating patients with histological evidence of recurrent PBC with ursodeoxycholic acid. As anticipated, there is biochemical improvement although it is too early to look for evidence of histological improvement.

SUMMARY

PBC remains a common indication for liver transplantation; indications and timing of the procedure are now well established. The short-term survival is usually excellent, with many centers reporting 5-year survival in excess of 70%. However, the disease recurs in the allograft in a small proportion of patients; whether this is of any clinical significance and the factors which predict recurrence remain to be established.

References

1. Neuberger J. Primary biliary cirrhosis. Lancet 1997;350:875–9.
2. European Liver Transplant Registry, Paris, 1997.

3. Jalan R, Lombard M. Patients with PBC have central but no peripheral fatigue. Hepatology 1996;24:167A(abstract).
4. Sorensen HT, Thulstrup A, Frijs S, et al. Cancer risk in patients with liver cirrhosis: a registry study based on 85000 person years. J Hepatol 1997;26(Suppl 1):100(abstract).
5. Michel J, Suc B, Montpeyroux F, et al. Liver reaction or transplantation for hepatocellular carcinoma? J Hepatol 1997;26:1274–80.
6. Penn I. The effect of immunosuppression on pre-existing cancers. Transplantation 1993; 55:742–7.
7. Shapiro J, Smith H, Schaffner F. Serum bilirubin: a prognostic factor in primary biliary cirrhosis. Gut 1979;20:137–40.
8. Christensen E. Prognostic models in chronic liver disease: validity, usefulness and future role. J Hepatol 1997;26:1414–24.
9. Dickson E, Grambsch P, Fleming T, Fisher L, Langworthy A. Prognosis for primary biliary cirrhosis: a model for decision making. Hepatology 1989;10:1–7.
10. Christensen E, Guson B, Neuberger J. Optimal timing of liver transplantation for patients with primary biliary cirrhosis: use of prognostic modelling. Gut 1997;41(suppl 3): A77(abstract).
11. Ransford R, Gunson B, Mayer A, Neuberger J. Analysis of patients dying on the liver transplant adult waiting list. Gut 1997;41(suppl 3):A239(abstract).
12. Neuberger J. Transplantation for primary biliary cirrhosis. Semin Liver Dis 1997;17:137–46.
13. Farges O, Saliba F, Farhamant H, et al. The incidence of rejection and infection after liver transplantation as a function of the primary disease: possible influence of alcohol and polyclonal immunoglobulins. Hepatology 1996;23:240–8.
14. Mor E, Solomon E, Gibbs J, et al. Acute cellular rejection following liver transplantation: clinical pathologic features and effect on outcome. Semin Liver Dis 1992;12:28–40.
15. Adams D. Mechanisms of liver allograft rejection in man. Clin Sci 1990;78:343–50.
16. Candinas D, Gunson B, Nightingale P, Hubscher S, McMaster P, Neuberger J. Sex mismatch as a risk factor for chronic rejection of liver allografts. Lancet 1995;346:1117–21.
17. Navasa M, Forms X, Sanchez V, et al. Quality of life, major medical complications and hospital service utilization in patients with primary biliary cirrhosis after liver transplantation. J Hepatol 1996;25:129–34.
18. Klein R, Huizenga J, Gips C, Berg P. Antimitochondrial antibody profiles in patients with primary biliary cirrhosis before orthotopic liver transplantation and titers of antimitochondrial antibody subtypes after liver transplantation. J Hepatol 1994;20:787–9.
19. Neuberger J, Portmann B, MacDougall B, Caine R, Williams R. Recurrence of primary biliary cirrhosis. N Engl J Med 1982;306:1–4.
20. Polson R, Portman B, Neuberger J, Caine R, Williams R. Evidence for disease recurrence after liver transplantation for primary biliary cirrhosis. Gastroenterology 1989;97:715–25.
21. Lerut J, Zimmerman A, Geretsch P, et al. Chronic rejection and extra-hepatic biliary obstruction 8 years after liver transplantation with gall bladder conduit. HPB Surgery 1991;18:173–84.
22. Buist L, Hubscher S, Vickers C, Michell I, Neuberger J, McMaster P. Does liver transplantation cure primary biliary cirrhosis? Transplant Proc 1989;21:2402.
23. Hubscher S, Elias E, Buckels J, McMaster P, Neuberger J. Primary biliary cirrhosis: histological evidence of recurrent disease after liver transplantation. J Hepatol 1993;18:173–84.
24. Demetris A, Markus B, Esquivel C, et al. Pathologic analysis of liver transplantation for primary biliary cirrhosis. Hepatology 1988;8:937–47.
25. Abu-Elmagd K, Demetris J, Rakela J, et al. Transplantation for primary biliary cirrhosis. Hepatology 1997;26:176A(abstract).
26. Gouw A, Haagsma E, Manns M, Klompmaker I, Slooff M, Gerber M. Is there recurrence of primary biliary cirrhosis after liver transplantation? J Hepatol 1994;20:500–7.
27. Ferrell L, Lee R, Brixko C, et al. Hepatic granulomas following liver transplantation. Transplantation 1995;60:926–33.
28. Dmitrewski J, Hubscher S, Mayer A, Neuberger J. Recurrence of primary biliary cirrhosis in the liver allograft: the effect of immunosuppression. J Hepatol 1996;24:253–7.
29. Yoshida E, Singh R, Vartarian R, Owen D. Late recurrent post-transplant primary biliary cirrhosis in British Columbia. Can J Gastroenterol 1997;11:229–31.
30. Mazariegos G, Reyes J, Marino I, et al. Weaning of immunosuppression in liver transplant recipients. Transplantation 1997;63:243–9.

31. Balan V, Batts K, Porayko M, Krom R, Ludwig J, Wiesner R. Histological evidence for recurrence of primary biliary cirrhosis after liver transplantation. Hepatology 1993; 18:1392–8.
32. Dietze D, Vogel W, Margreiter R. Primary biliary cirrhosis (PBC) after liver transplantation. Transplant Proc 1990;22:1501–2.
33. Sebagh M, Farges O, Dubel L, Samuel D, Bismuth H, Reynes M. Recurrence of primary biliary cirrhosis (PBC) after liver transplantation: the risk is real. J Hepatol 1996; 24(suppl 1):125(abstract).

20
New clinical trials in primary biliary cirrhosis: design and endpoints

J. EVERHART

INTRODUCTION

During the last 30 years, clinical trial methodology has evolved from the interface of epidemiology, biostatistics, and clinical medicine to a specialty with its own experts, terminology, computer programs, books, and journals. During much of this time, randomized clinical trials for the treatment of primary biliary cirrhosis (PBC) were being conducted[1-5]. This chapter discusses three important issues in the design of therapeutic trials of PBC: choice of the primary research issue, sample size and power calculations, and choice of the primary response variable. It is hoped that consideration of these issues will result in well-planned trials in PBC and will serve a note of caution to investigators before embarking on a trial that may not be capable of achieving its goal.

ASSUMPTIONS

To help focus the discussion on new trials in PBC, several assumptions will be made regarding aspects of design. First, the discussion will pertain to randomized controlled clinical trials of PBC. This approach requires randomized and concurrent treatment assignment of at least two groups of patients. Comparison with an historical cohort cannot be the focus of such a trial. Nevertheless, comparison of trial outcomes with outcomes in other groups of patients can be important in demonstrating the validity and generalizability of the trial results. Second, discussion will be limited to studies in which intervention is directed against the liver disease of PBC. Trials directed purely at the consequences of PBC, such as osteoporosis and pruritus, will not be discussed. Third, it will be assumed that a new intervention will be compared in some way with an existing standard, currently the bile acid ursodeoxycholic acid, also called ursodiol. Also, the new intervention can be, but does not have to be, combined with ursodiol. Combination makes sense when the intervention under consideration has a different mechanism of action from ursodiol. For example, a new intervention might primarily have anti-inflammatory properties or inhibit fibrosis. Fourth, the new intervention should not be so obviously effective as to eliminate the need for a comparison with standard therapy. A drug that directly targets the etiology of the disease resulting in complete reversal of the disease process would be such an intervention. Unfortunately, based on current knowledge, it is unlikely that such an agent will become available for at least several years. Finally, only efficacy trials will be considered. These are trials of such rigor and size that their results will give primary guidance as to whether an intervention will be used in clinical practice. In the regulatory approval process, the United States Food and Drug Administration terms such studies Phase 3 trials.

WHAT IS THE QUESTION?

Investigators planning a clinical trial need to agree on a primary study question. Having an overriding goal simplifies planning and execution and helps to keep costs down. For a chronic liver disease such as PBC, such a goal might involve the effectiveness of a new drug and could, for example, be stated as follows: "Does the new drug decrease the number of deaths and liver transplantations compared with standard therapy?" This primary study question is the one the investigators are most interested in. It should be clinically meaningful based on an outcome that all would agree is of importance. It is also the question on which sample size and study duration are based.

Most clinical trials also have secondary questions. Other outcomes, such as quality of life deterioration or liver disease decompensation, might complement a study with death or transplantation as the primary response variable. Investigators often wish to know if therapy is effective in a particular subgroup of patients, though rarely is sample size large enough to provide a firm answer. These secondary response variables and subgroup analyses should be specified in advance. Post-hoc analyses are fraught with potential biases from deriving and testing hypotheses after seeing the data. Other secondary questions can be answered through ancillary studies, which may involve more technically complex or expensive measures on a subset of patients. Ancillary studies should not be undertaken that adversely affect study adherence, retention, or outcome.

SAMPLE SIZE

Most studies that have reported 'negative' findings have not had adequate power to detect an important clinical effect of an intervention. For example, in a review of 71 published randomized controlled clinical trials that did not find significant differences between groups, it was found that 50 of the trials had a greater than 10% chance of missing a 50% improvement[6]. Sample size calculations are an essential part of planning randomized clinical trials designed to determine drug efficacy. Because trials of PBC are costly and lengthy, it would be inappropriate to commit significant resources to a trial that is unlikely to determine if a therapy is effective. Although sample size calculations are a necessary part of planning a trial, there is a number of reasons why they are approximations. First, the most important parameters used to estimate sample size are the event rates in the treatment arms. These rates are usually derived from small studies or studies in populations different from the study population and thus can be imprecise. Second, researchers often exaggerate the presumed effectiveness of a new treatment, assuming a more substantial difference in event rates when preliminary data suggest less of a difference. Third, even when the event rate is as expected in the treatment group, controls often have better outcomes than anticipated, reducing the expected difference. Finally, the mathematical models used to determine sample size only approximate the distribution of the study outcome. Because of these vagaries of sample size calculations, it has been suggested that it is better to overestimate sample size and possibly terminate the trial early than to extend it[7]. However, in some slowly progressive diseases such as PBC, a difference in response may be apparent only after many years of therapy. Thus, planning the trial for a long duration at the outset may be better than focusing solely on a larger sample size, which may be difficult to accrue in such a relatively uncommon disease.

CHOICE OF RESPONSE VARIABLES

Perhaps the most important issue in planning a clinical trial of PBC is the choice of the primary response variable or endpoint. An important clinical outcome, such as death or transplantation, would be most desirable, but requires a large and lengthy trial. Listing for transplantation has been suggested as an alternative to transplantation. Reasons for proposing listing for transplantation over actual transplantation as a primary response variable include an earlier outcome and because non-disease-related factors influence time of transplantation. But non-disease factors also determine time of listing. For example, transplant candidates with type O blood are known to wait longer for transplantation than candidates with other blood types. As a result, transplant centers have listed patients with type O blood when healthier. By the time of transplantation, clinical differences between blood types have resolved[8]. Patient decompensation might be an alternative to liver transplantation or death. However, there is a number of ways to decompensate, perhaps not all of equal importance or measurable in a standardized and systematic manner. The alternative to a clinical response is an intermediate or 'surrogate' response variable, such as change in serum bilirubin concentration or liver histological stage. These response variables may be observed more quickly and with a smaller sample size, but the clinical importance is not clear. They are discussed in detail below.

The remainder of this chapter concerns the practical consequences of choosing a response variable. These choices are the clinical endpoint of death or liver transplantation and the surrogate endpoints of increase in serum bilirubin concentration or development of cirrhosis. The starting

Table 1 Large multicenter randomized controlled clinical trials of ursodiol in the treatment of primary biliary cirrhosis

Investigator	Location	Sample size	Duration (years)	Response variables
Heathcote et al.[9]	Canada, multicenter	222	2–4	50% decrease in bilirubin rise
Poupon et al.[10]	France, multicenter	146	2–4	Disease progression
Lindor et al.[11]	US, multicenter	180	4	Disease progression
Combes et al.[12]	US, multicenter	151	2	Disease progression

point will be the 4 largest trials of ursodiol in the treatment of PBC (Table 1). These are discussed from a different perspective by Dr. Carithers in Chapter 18. One point to be noted is the size of the studies: 146 to 222 patients enrolled through multicenter regional and national efforts. Second, the duration of therapy was 2–4 years and third, the primary response variables concerned disease progression. Fourth, only one of the trials defined disease progression using a single measurement: the Canadian trial, which examined serum bilirubin rise. The other trials defined disease progression with as many as 9 different clinical parameters. With so many response variables, it becomes more difficult to determine an appropriate sample size, obtain all outcome measurements, and interpret the results.

The results of three studies have been combined to examine whether ursodiol prolongs the time until death or transplantation[13]. Data from individual patients were combined, which allowed the authors to examine outcomes among subsets of patients. The results of this combined analysis may be useful in planning new analyses. First, the overall transplantation-free survival at four years was slightly less than 80% for the ursodiol-treated patients (Figure 1). Such results, adjusted for disease severity, can be used to estimate survival in new trials that use ursodiol in one of the treatment arms. Second, the effects of ursodiol were observed in subgroups of serum bilirubin (Figure 2) and histological stage (Figure 3). In the subgroup analysis of bilirubin, the 4-year transplantation-free survival of patients assigned ursodiol was > 85% if their serum bilirubin concentration was ≤ 1.4 mg/dl, about 80% for bilirubin between 1.4 and 3.5 mg/dl, and about 35% for bilirubin > 3.5 mg/dl. Transplant-free survival was about 85% for ursodiol-treated patients with histological stages 1 and 2, about 75% for stage 3 and < 65% for stage 4. In addition to being useful for planning new trials, these subgroup results illustrate a problem that new therapeutic trials must address: a new therapy may be most effective in preventing progression in patients with lower serum bilirubin concentrations or at earlier histological stage, but excellent transplantation-free survival in these groups will make it difficult to show a survival benefit of a new therapy.

The effect of using ursodiol on trial design can be shown through an actual example. A trial sponsored by the National Institute of Diabetes and Digestive and Kidney Diseases, called the PBC ursodiol and methotrexate or placebo study (PUMPS), has randomized patients to ursodiol and oral methotrexate or to ursodiol and placebo after at least a six-month run-in

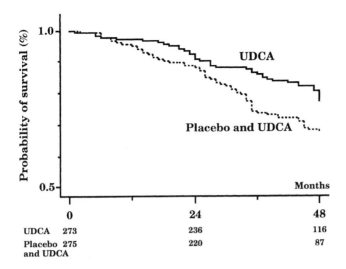

Figure 1 Probability of survival free of liver transplantation according to the initial randomization. This probability was significantly greater in the patients treated for 4 years with UDCA than in those who first received placebo and then UDCA ($p < 0.001$; relative risk, 1.92; 95% confidence interval, 1.30–2.82). (Reproduced from ref. 20)

period on ursodiol. Twelve US centers began randomizing patients in January 1994.

Power calculations have been performed to plan study duration based on the following assumptions: a total of 260 patients randomized equally to the two treatment arms, an exponential survival (rates of death and transplantation increase with study duration), and use of a two-sided log rank test at a significance level of 0.05 (Emerson S, personal communication). One example of the power calculations is shown in Figure 4 for an assumed 5-year 70% transplant-free survival in the ursodiol/placebo arm against a 5-year survival in the ursodiol/methotrexate arm of 85% (hazard ratio of 2.19 for ursodiol/placebo vs. ursodiol/methotrexate), 83% (hazard ratio of 1.91) and 81% (hazard ratio of 1.69). With survival of 85% in the ursodiol/ methotrexate arm, the study would take approximately 4.5 years to achieve a power of 80% and 6.0 years to achieve a power of 90%. This means that, at 6 years, if the actual 5-year survival were 85% in the ursodiol/methotrexate arm and 70% in the ursodiol/placebo arm, the study would have a 90% chance of detecting a difference in the two arms at $p = 0.05$ and a 10% chance of failing to detect such a difference. If the actual 5-year survival in the ursodiol/methotrexate arm was 83%, then it would take nearly 6.5 years to achieve a power of 80% and more than 8 years to achieve a power of 90%. If the 5-year survival were 81% in the combined treatment arm, then the trial duration would need to continue well beyond 8 years to achieve an 80% power.

If the actual 5-year survival in the ursodiol/placebo arm were 80%, then the 5-year survival in the ursodiol/methotrexate arm would need to be at least 90% to achieve a power of 80% within 8 years (not shown).

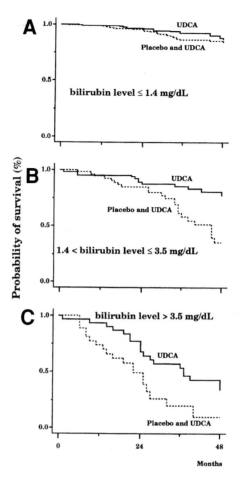

Figure 2 Probability of survival free of liver transplantation in the original UDCA group and the original placebo group in three subgroups defined by three baseline serum bilirubin levels ([A], <1.4 mg/dL; [B], 1.4–3.5 mg/dL; and [C], >3.5 mg/dL). There was no significant difference between the two treatment groups for the (A) low-risk subgroup ($p = 0.16$), whereas the difference was significant for the (B) medium-risk and (C) high-risk groups ($p < 0.001$ and $p < 0.03$, respectively). (Reproduced from ref. 20)

Thus, in a trial of a new therapy being compared with ursodiol, even if the new therapy is highly effective, the study needs to be carried out on many patients for a long duration. Even with recruiting more patients than any other trial in the modern era of liver transplantation, the trial described here will need to continue longer than any other recent trials to have a reasonable chance of detecting a substantial treatment effect if death and liver transplantation are used as the primary response variables.

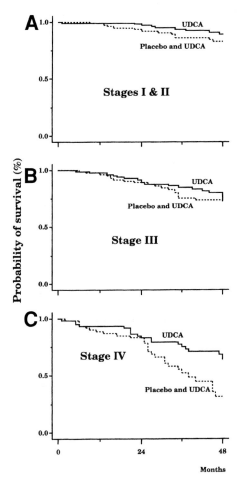

Figure 3 Probability of survival free of liver transplantation in three subgroups according to histological stage at entry; stages I and II, stage III, and stage IV. There was no significant difference between the two treatment groups for histological (A) stages I and II and (B) stage III subgroups ($p = 0.06$ and $p = 0.66$, respectively), whereas the difference was significant for the (C) stage IV subgroup ($p < 0.01$). (Reproduced from ref. 20)

SURROGATE RESPONSE VARIABLES

Because of the difficulty in observing a treatment effect on transplant-free survival, surrogate response variables may be considered as alternatives. These are variables that are thought to predict clinically important events, but do not directly affect the health of the patient. Surrogate response variables are appealing because they may allow for considerably smaller and shorter trials. Surrogate response variables are also useful in the early stages of trial development, such as determining the appropriate dose of drug to use in a larger study. However, for a surrogate response variable to be used in an efficacy trial, it should meet several criteria. First, it should

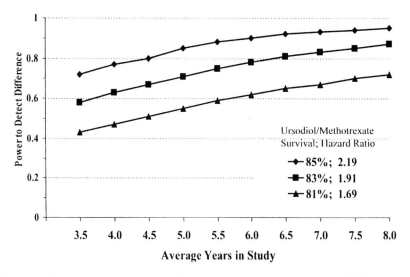

Figure 4 Estimated power to detect difference in transplant-free survival of 70% between ursodiol/placebo-treated patients and 81%, 83%, and 85% in ursodiol/methotrexate-treated patients.

truly reflect clinical outcome. This criterion requires that the surrogate variable be highly correlated with the clinical outcome. Beyond correlation, the surrogate should reflect the biological process of the disease such that the surrogate should be· in the causal pathway between early disease and poor clinical outcome. An understanding of the causal pathway requires extensive investigation into the pathophysiology of the disease and its natural history. Second, a surrogate response variable needs to be assessed reliably and accurately. Third, the surrogate should not be so intrusive as to discourage patient participation nor so expensive as to negate the cost savings of a smaller trial. Fourth, the trial must still be sufficiently large to detect important adverse events. Finally, the results of a trial using a surrogate response variable must be acceptable to the medical community.

Serum bilirubin concentration could be considered as a laboratory example of a surrogate response variable. Serum bilirubin can be obtained accurately and reliably. Plus, it is highly correlated with survival; in the combined ursodiol analysis, low baseline serum bilirubin concentration was the most potent predictor of transplant-free survival[13]. However, it remains to be shown whether the serum bilirubin concentration of patients treated with ursodiol is as strong a predictor of survival as in patients not treated with ursodiol. One way to examine this issue would be to determine if the subsequent survival of patients after 6 months of therapy with ursodiol is similar to the survival of patients with comparable levels of bilirubin prior to ursodiol treatment. Because of ursodiol's choleretic effect, it would be required in all arms in any treatment comparison if serum bilirubin concentration were to be used as a primary response variable. Also, it is not clear to what extent serum bilirubin is merely a marker for disease progression or is actually in the causal pathway to liver failure. The answer to this problem should largely determine whether serum bilirubin or any other laboratory measurement would be acceptable to the medical community as a primary response variable.

Liver histology represents another type of surrogate response variable. If cirrhosis were used as the primary response variable, it would clearly be in the causal pathway to endstage liver disease, leading to death or transplantation. Cirrhosis is also a stable condition and not known to be reversible. However, there are several problems in using cirrhosis as a response variable. First, the effect of therapy on patients who already have cirrhosis could not be evaluated. Such patients constituted 25% of patients in the combined analysis[13]. Second, liver biopsy is subject to measurement error because of small tissue samples and observer variation among pathologists. The resulting measurement error may be one reason for the relatively poor predictive value of histological stage on transplant-free survival in the combined analysis. Third, because liver biopsy is an invasive procedure, complete outcome data would become difficult to obtain, particularly in a study of several years that might require several biopsies of each patient.

CONCLUSION

This chapter has focused on the choice of primary response variables and the effect on sample size in potential efficacy trials of PBC. Trials that are designed to show a survival benefit from a new therapy are likely to require many patients, last for many years, and require considerable resources and dedication to complete. Thus, a great deal of thought and preparation should go into planning a trial that will answer the study question. Surrogate measures allow for smaller, shorter, and less-expensive trials. However, current surrogates appear too crude to accurately measure disease progression or could potentially respond to therapy without changing the course of the disease. Trials will become easier to perform with increased knowledge of pathogenesis and disease progression.

References

1. Heathcote J, Ross A, Sherlock S. A prospective controlled trial of azathioprine in primary biliary cirrhosis. Gastroenterology 1976;70(5):656–60.
2. Dickson ER, Fleming TR, Wiesner RH, et al. Trial of penicillamine in advanced primary biliary cirrhosis. N Engl J Med 1985;312(16):1011–15.
3. Neuberger J, Christensen E, Portmann B, et al. Double blind controlled trial of d-penicillamine in patients with primary biliary cirrhosis. Gut 1985;26(2):114–19.
4. Bodenheimer H Jr, Schaffner F, Pezzullo J. Evaluation of colchicine therapy in primary biliary cirrhosis. Gastroenterology 1988;95(1):124–9.
5. Kaplan MM, Alling DW, Zimmerman HJ, et al. A prospective trial of colchicine for primary biliary cirrhosis. N Engl J Med 1986;315(23):1448–54.
6. Frieman JA, Chalmers TC, Smith H Jr, Kuebler RR. The importance of beta, the type II error and sample size in the design and interpretation of the randomized control trial: survey of 71 "negative" trials. N Engl J Med 1978;299:690–4.
7. Friedman LM, Furberg CD, DeMets DL. Fundamentals of Clinical Trials, 3rd edn. St. Louis, MO: Mosby-Year Book Inc.; 1996:361.
8. Everhart JE, Lombardero M, Detre KM, et al. Increased waiting time for liver transplantation results in higher mortality. Transplantation. 1997;64(9):1300–6.

9. Heathcote EJ, Cauch-Dudek K, Walker V, *et al.* The Canadian Multicenter Double-blind Randomized Controlled Trial of ursodeoxycholic acid in primary biliary cirrhosis. A randomized, double-blind, placebo-controlled trial of ursodeoxycholic acid in primary biliary cirrhosis. Hepatology 1995;22(3):759–66.
10. Poupon RE, Poupon R, Balkau B. Ursodiol for the long-term treatment of primary biliary cirrhosis. The UDCA–PBC Study Group. N Engl J Med 1994;330(19):1342–7.
11. Lindor KD, Dickson ER, Jorgensen RA, *et al.* The combination of ursodeoxycholic acid and methotrexate for patients with primary biliary cirrhosis: the results of a pilot study. Hepatology 1995;22(4):1158–62.
12. Combes B, Carithers RL Jr, Maddrey WC, *et al.* A randomized, double-blind placebo-controlled trial of ursodeoxycholic acid in primary biliary cirrhosis. Hepatology 1995; 22(3):759–60.
13. Poupon RE, Lindor KD, Cauch-Dudek K, Dickson ER, Poupon R, Heathcote EJ. Combined analysis of randomized controlled trials of ursodeoxycholic acid in primary biliary cirrhosis. Gastroenterology 1997;113(3):884–90.

Index